(*Euterpe oleracea*)

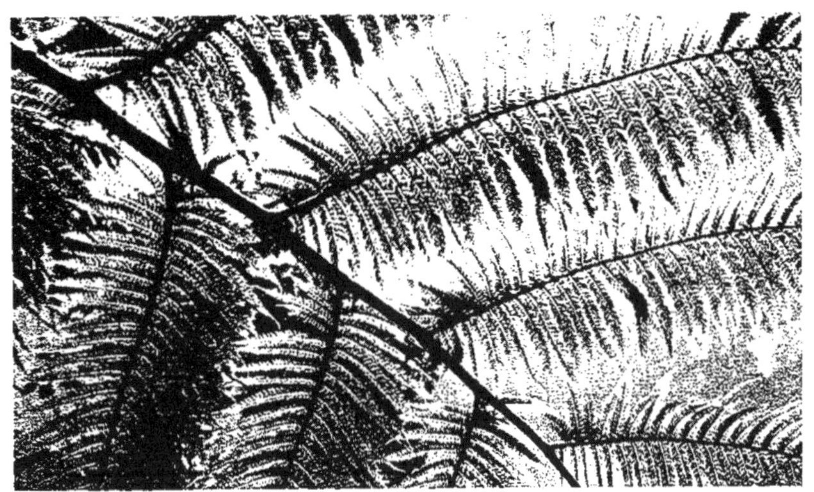

An Extraordinary Antioxidant-Rich Palm Fruit

Alexander G. Schauss, PhD, FACN

Biosocial Publications
Tacoma, WA

Acai (Euterpe oleracea): An Extraordinary Antioxidant-Rich Palm Fruit

First Edition (October, 2006)
Second Edition (November, 2006)

Manufactured in the United States

ISBN 0-943685-30-3

Library of Congress Cataloging-in-Publication Date

Schauss, Alexander 1948 -

Biosocial Publications
P.O. Box 1174
Tacoma, WA 98401

Disclaimer:

This work on acai fruit is not intended to be an exhaustive or scholarly technical work. The intention of this book is to provide the public with some useful information on the subject given the increasing interest in acai fruit now that it is being consumed beyond a few South American countries.

The reader should not interpret any of the information in this book as medical advice. If you believe you have a symptom, condition or disease, always consult a licensed health care practitioner or physician.

CONTENTS

Introduction

In the late 1960's, while pursuing a major in history at the University of New Mexico (UNM) in Albuquerque, I explored a region of southern New Mexico called the Membres Valley on weekends. A combination of research and luck resulted in my discovering the remains of a long lost tribe of Mimbres Indians whose culture flourished in the Membres Valley of what is now New Mexico and then disappeared without leaving any written record.

The discovery led to my induction into Phi Alpha Theta, the national honorary society in history, during my sophomore year. Truth be known, while searching for any evidence of their previous existence within a 25 square mile area, I chased a butterfly that just seemed out of place in the desert for nearly a quarter of a mile, alongside the dirt road I had parked my car to read a map. That butterfly literally took me right to a spring in the middle of the desert. There along side a pool of water I found a piece of pottery that had some paintings of animal figures. I took a few pieces back to a professor who taught New Mexico history at UNM, and well, the rest is history.

It turned out the Mimbres Indians left the Membres Valley when over 25 miles of the river that ran through it into what is now southern New Mexico and Mexico dried up after a period of prolonged drought. Yet it mysteriously reappears to this day approximately 25 miles south of what is now the US-Mexico border. Possibly the Mimbres moved south, or headed west for the Mogollon Mountains that today is part of the Gila National Forest, or possibly resettled north along the Rio Grande River. No one knows to this day where the Mimbres Indians resettled or if they perished.

The following summer, I had the opportunity to take a sociology course at City University of New York (CUNY) in upper Manhattan. To meet a course requirement, involving field research, I was given the opportunity to study a theory I had involving the use of very high doses of ascorbic acid (vitamin C). To test my theory I was allowed to work with a population of heroin addicts just a few blocks from the CUNY campus near Columbia University. My research project led to the development of a protocol for the treatment of withdrawal symptoms associated with withdrawing from an addiction to heroin. Basically, my research showed that if an addict hooked on heroin is given enough ascorbic acid, dissolved in water or juice throughout the day, they could withdraw from their addiction without experiencing side effects, a brutal and painful treatment regime known in those days as "going cold turkey." Many of the addicts also were reported to have recovered from hepatitis A, a viral infection.

It was my first exposure to the health benefits of using an antioxidant. (Later the therapeutic effectiveness of this protocol was confirmed by the National Institute on Drug Abuse (NIDA). They came to Seattle, Washington, where some years later I was the research director of the Institute for Biosocial Research in the graduate school of City University. During their visit they observed the treatment administered by the county's addiction treatment services director, Dr. Janice Keller-Phelps, MD. Dr. Keller-Phelps described the treatment method as if it was "a cure for cancer for addicts." Had she not previously worked for the NIDA, and been a medical director of another government agency in Maryland, they probably would not have given the treatment the level of interest it received. Four days of interviews with heroin addicts living in King County, Washington, who went through the treatment, led them to share their amazement at the effectiveness of this "orthomolecular" treatment. The term "orthomolecular" was coined by two-time Nobel Laureate, Dr. Linus Pauling, a noted chemist, who won Nobel prizes in chemistry and peace.

The results were so profound that it attracted the attention of Dr. Linus Pauling. Meeting Dr. Pauling also led to the publication of my first book. On the cover of that work appeared Dr. Pauling's signature, along with a quote from him on the importance of using the right molecules of compounds naturally found in nature to prevent and treat afflictions experienced by humans. As my first work dealt with the field of behavioral sciences, Dr. Pauling wrote the following statement on the cover:

> "Orthomolecular treatment is the achievement and preservation of good mental health by provision of the optimum molecular environment for the mind, especially the optimum concentration of substances normally present in the human body, such as the vitamins."

A few years later, in 1983, I was invited to give a series of lectures on research I had conducted before the McCarrison Society's European Conference on Nutrition and Behavior held on the campus of Oxford University. Among some 200 attendees from institutions such as Oxford University, Cambridge University, the University of Reading, the University of London, was a special guest and then newly-elected President of the Society, Professor Hugh McDonald Sinclair. Knighted by Queen Elizabeth, Sir Hugh Sinclair earned degrees in animal physiology at Oriel College, Oxford, and later taught biochemistry at Oxford, and was a "Senior Demy" at Oxford's medical school, Magdalen College. He also completed studies in medicine at the University College Hospital Medical School in London, where he subsequently became a Lecturer in Physiology at University College, London. Most people in England know him for serving as Winston Churchill's advisor on nutrition and war-time Minister of Food, during World War II. A few years after the war, Dr. Sinclair was awarded the U.S. Presidential Medal of Freedom and made an honorary Brigadier General of the British Army.

Born in 1910, Professor Sinclair became one of the 20th century's outstanding experts in human nutrition, widely known for claiming that what he called "diseases of civilization" such as coronary heart disease, cancer, diabetes, inflammation, strokes and skin disease, are worsened by "bad fats."

Through subsequent invitations to return to Oxford immediately following my presentation before the McCarrison Society, and the publication of my lectures in a British nutrition journal, and review in the *Sunday London Times*, Dr. Sinclair invited me to return to Oxford and live there to teach a course with Professor Joseph Egger, MD, who held joint professorships at both the University of London and the University of Munich. This gave me the opportunity to live in Oxford with my family and spend time with Professor Sinclair in his remarkable home in Sutton Courtenay (just outside of Oxford), were he maintained one of the most remarkable private libraries I have ever seen anywhere in the world.

The opportunity of living in Oxford and soaking in the knowledge that permeates this great institution of higher learning proved to turn my attention more and more towards the study of ethnobotany. Professor Sinclair shared with me his field research in the arctic where he lived wholly on the diet consumed by native Inuits. Documenting the effects of living on an Inuit diet on his health in remarkable detail led to the recognition of the importance of what are known as long-chain fatty acids found in fish oils and their effect on the clogging (aggregation) of blood platelets and thus the incidence of thrombosis, a common disease known to developed civilizations.

The course Dr. Egger and I taught was offered through the Department of Pediatrics at The John Radcliffe Hospital in Oxford. What made living and teaching in Oxford particularly exciting was having a library card that provided access to Oxford University's Radcliffe Library. There, I could examine a remarkable collection of historical works on nutrition. This included accounts written hundreds of years earlier by British explorers and naturalists describing the food habits of native populations around the world. These marvelous accounts led to fascinating discussions with Professor Sinclair.

It was during one of our meetings that I mentioned an experience I had in 1980 during a visit to Australia to lecture at the University of New South Wales. I had just arrived in Sydney after completing the first phase of field research studying the cause of Guamanian Parkinson's disease in Guam, a remote Pacific Island. Unfortunately, I had caught a nasty cold just as I left Guam and by noon of the following day hours before my lecture that evening, my temperature had risen to 105 degrees Fahrenheit. I was becoming weaker by the minute. My host, a naturopathic physician based in Sydney, called Dr. Archie Kalokerinos, MD, who was using vitamin C to treat Aboriginal infants reacting to childhood vaccinations. Prior to his using vitamin C, one in every two Aboriginal children given vaccinations and immunizations died, until he discovered that a single one gram injection of vitamin C administered a week before hand would prevent all deaths. His book, *Every Second Child*, is a fascinating account of his discovery.

Upon his arrival, Dr. Kalokineros hooked me up to an intravenous (IV) drip of ascorbic acid (pure vitamin C). Over the course of a few hours my temperature dropped. By 6 pm that evening my temperature was 99 degrees and

I felt a surge of energy. That evening I started my lecture promptly at 7:30 pm and lectured straight through to 10 pm. I still recall how remarkably clear my mind was that evening, particularly my recall of literature I had read.

Professor Sinclair and Dr. Kalokineros advocated restricting the intake of excessive amounts of refined carbohydrates. This did not endear Professor Sinclair in particular with the World Sugar Council, based in London, or its allies in the food industry who put sugar into so many foods to make them more appealing given the genetic propensity we have towards sweet tasting foods (e.g. carbonated cola beverages, children's cereals, some of which were over 50% refined sugar). Sinclair predicted that the world would suffer from an epidemic of obesity by eating foods low in nutritional density, which he referred to as causing "overconsumption malnutrition." He passed away in 1990, but his beliefs are now being accepted by more nutritional experts as one of the root causes of the epidemic of obesity seen around the world today.

But among Sinclair's many skills was his ability to teach others how to think and use the power of observation.

These seemingly unrelated experiences in New Mexico, New York City, Oxford, and Sydney, helped me to recognize the existence of a food that we've now discovered has the highest antioxidant activity of any fruit or vegetable found in the world. I think of these mentors much like that butterfly that led me to discover the site of the Mimbres Indians in the desert of southern New Mexico. Without their guidance I might never have been able to realize the importance of studying a relatively unknown fruit growing in a palm tree in the Amazon, that led to years of research and the writing of this book.

Besides the good fortune of meeting so many great minds around the world, I also needed to have a foundation through years of working with botanicals to understand the forces that make plants produce compounds called "antioxidants." But we're getting ahead of ourselves. So before delving straight into what we know about acai today, I need to share just one more experience.

On one of my trips to Europe I had the fortune of stopping in the town of Coimbra in central Portugal. This historical city is the home of the second oldest university in the world, the University of Coimbra, founded in 1290 by King Dinis. The University sits on a hill above Avenida Emidio Navarro, which runs parallel to the Mondego River (Rio Mondego). Hiking up the narrow cobble stone streets to the university's central square is an experience itself.

Desiring to do some research in the library of the University's Anthropology Museum and Laboratory, Faculty of Sciences and Technology, one of the department's faculty invited me to view a remarkable and priceless display of ancient Amazonian masks kept in a secured area of the museum not open to the public. Among the many masks on display were those of the now extinct Jurupixuna Indians who had lived in the Orinoco basin of Brazil. The Jurupixunas perished shortly after making contact with European explorers who found their settlements in the late 18th century.

Early accounts by Portuguese Europeans exploring the region known today as Amazonia in Brasil (the Portuguese spelling for Brazil) described the use of masks worn during dances honoring the birth of a child or a marriage, to recognize a successful hunting expedition, or to celebrate the completion of the season's harvest of a palm fruit. A palm fruit? Yes, a palm fruit.

This information, recorded by explorers centuries ago, supported the concept that in the Amazon were foods with unusual properties. A fruit that had extraordinary attributes, possibly unlike any food in the world.

Unfortunately, with the arrival of European explorers and settlers to the Western hemisphere there also came many diseases such as small pox for which the native population possessed no immunity. As these diseases spread from village to village, thousands would die, their immune systems unable to repel the contagious pathogens responsible for their suffering.

It was only in the late 20th century that scientists realized that foods not only possessed nutrients and calories, but also contained phytochemicals that could be equally as important as vitamins and minerals in contributing to our health. Some natural chemicals found in plants are able to prevent, mitigate or treat diseases or afflictions. We now recognize that our forests, plains, coastlines and jungles, hold a literal pharmacy of compounds that are produced by tens of thousands of terrestrial plant species and marine plants and organisms.

Anthropologists and historians are certain that ancient people gave thanks to the their gods or spirits for the bounty nature provided them. But for a palm fruit?

Among over 2,000 species of palms growing around the world, only a few provide a fruit that humans consume. Two well-known examples of palm fruits are coconuts and dates. But neither is found in the Amazon. So which palm fruit might the natives of the Amazon have celebrated?

I had a clue – an edible palm fruit only found in Amazonia and two related species growing at higher elevations.

That Amazonian palm tree is known to botanists by its Latin name, *Euterpe oleracea*, and to natives as "acai" (pronounced, ah-sa-ee). Indications in the literature, based on some studies done in Brazil, described a class of compounds called polyphenols found in palm fruit. More important, there was no evidence that indicated anyone had done a systemic study of acai's chemistry or properties, beyond identifying its nutritional content (e.g., vitamins, minerals, etc).

Fortunately, I work at one of the world's leading natural products research institutes, AIBMR Life Sciences, as the company's lead scientist and Director of Natural and Medicinal Products Research. This gave me access to laboratories around the world to study the properties and characteristics of the acai fruit – that same fruit Amazonian tribes revered centuries ago and as I learned, remained a part of their culture to this day.

While beginning my studies I discovered that the pulp of the acai fruit had the highest level of antioxidant activity *in vitro* of any fruit or vegetable. In time it was also determined that the freeze-dried pulp of acai fruit had by far the highest antioxidant activity *in vitro* compared to other food drying methods (such as sun drying, spray drying, dehydration, or thin film drying).

Using reliable and validated methods for determining the oxygen radical absorbance capacity (ORAC) of a food, we looked at whether acai fruit had broad-spectrum antioxidant activity and were surprised to see it did, based on the peroxynitrite activity capacity assay (NORAC), hydroxyl radical oxygen activity capacity assay (HORAC) and superoxide radical absorbance capacity assay (SOD). We also found compounds in the freeze-dried fruit that helped direct us toward clinical studies that could confirm anecdotal reports of its health benefits.

Our body produces free radicals every second of our life. Just breathing causes them to appear, since we breathe in oxygen, which is used by our cell's energy producing mitochondria. When exercising free radicals are produced as a by-product, which is countered by antioxidants, some of which are produced in our body and not reliant upon what we eat, while others are dependent on what we eat. Excessive free radical production (oxidative stress) can have a very negative effect on our health. Eating certain fruits, vegetables and nuts, that are rich in antioxidants, can insure that our diet contains compounds that have free-radical scavenging activity.

Another way of understanding free radicals is to think of rust. Rust is caused by oxygen. The faster you rust, the faster you age. You see the effect of oxygen when you bite into an apple. Before long it turns brown due to an enzyme called polyphenol oxidase. Apply an anti-oxidant such as vitamin C solution onto the site where the apple was bitten, and you will see it stays white because it doesn't need to release the enzyme since vitamin C is doing the work for the apple. The only difference is the vitamin C does not cause a reaction that leaves a brownish color. Hence, an exogenous antioxidant can reduce the demand for an indigenous antioxidant. Our diet provides exogenous antioxidants.

Oxidative stress caused by free radicals has been identified as a major factor in the progression of aging and a contributor to numerous diseases. The role of "anti-oxidants" is to act like a sponge, mopping up or removing excessive oxygen radicals before they can harm healthy cells, but not to such an excessive degree that they could interfere with the benefits that free radicals provide, especially to the immune system in its effort to rid the body of pathogens, cells that have lost their ability to function, or cancer cells.

Could the natives that survived the diseases brought by the Europeans have benefited by consuming acai fruit? Could it have helped some of them survive? We might never know. But it certainly got me to thinking about the possibility.

Let's go back to my visit to Coimbra, Portugal. While there, I visited the department of anthropology at the University of Coimbra. This is the department that serves as curators of the masks brought back from Amazonia discussed earlier.

The university maintains a remarkable collection of books and manuscripts that are hundreds of years old. I arranged to meet one of the professors of anthropology to assist me in doing research in the department's library. I wondered if they had any knowledge of the whereabouts of hand drawings made by early Portuguese explorers showing natives harvesting, transporting, or consuming any palm fruits in Amazonia. Seconds after posing this question, the professor headed into the department's library and without hesitation found an oversized book that contained rare hand drawings made by an 18th century Portuguese explorer and naturalist. Only one other library in the world had these drawings, and it was in Lisbon, but these were different in that they did not show the background behind the natives, whereas the Coimbra book included it.

I watched the professor remove the book from the shelf with the greatest of care. She laid it down on the table and slowly opened its cover to reveal the title page. Every page thereafter revealed a remarkable series of drawings of Amazonian animals, fish, insects, and plants. Finally, we came upon some drawings of natives the explorers had encountered living near tributaries of the Amazon River.

There it was, the palm tree known to botanists by its Latin name, *Euterpe oleracea*. There was no question this was the acai palm, due to its distinctive long, pendulous fronds and narrow trunk. Here I stood, in one of the oldest libraries in the world looking at drawings made hundreds of years ago showing Amazonian natives harvesting and carrying baskets of acai fruit with the exact palm tree I was looking for in the background!

Before I left the university campus I learned that it was fortunate that I had not looked for this particular drawing in Lisbon, because I would not have seen the palm trees. For some unexplained reason, the drawing in Lisbon only showed exactly the same native holding a basket, but the background landscape was missing. There turned out to be two versions of the same drawing of this native, and the one in Coimbra included the background with the acai palm and its fruit. What luck!

Before leaving the university, I made arrangements to have both drawings photocopied for me to bring back to the United States. A picture of that native holding his basket with the fruit and the acai palms in the background is found in Figure 1.

As a scientist, I need to view data with objectivity. One would believe that there is a consensus among scientists, for example, that antioxidants found in foods will cure all diseases. Not everyone agrees with this premise. In fact there is a body of studies that disagrees with the premise that antioxidants will prevent

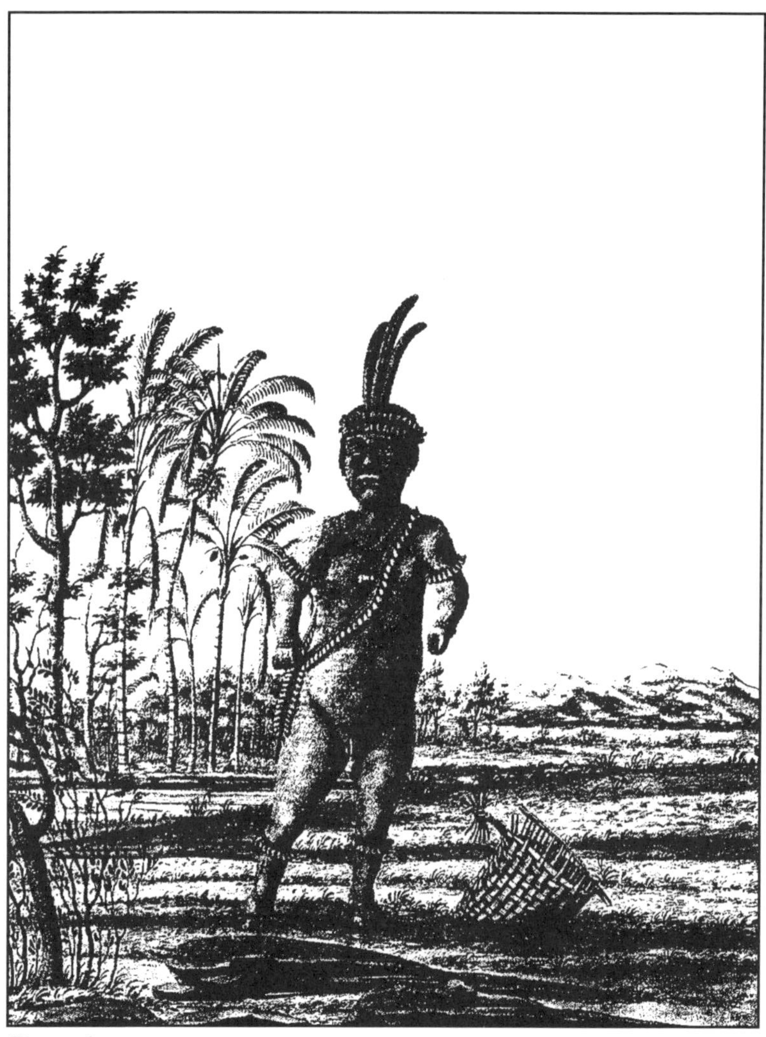

Figure 1

or treat diseases. Part of the reason there is such disagreement comes from just a few scientists. Recent studies are repudiating their claims as a vast body of science is documenting the benefits of antioxidants, particularly related to conditions and diseases associated with aging.

Fruits and vegetables rich in antioxidants contain hundreds of compounds. The evidence from population studies, a field called epidemiology, tells us that eating a diet rich in fruits and vegetables does contribute to a lower incidence of many diseases. The jury is out as to whether extracts of fruits and vegetables, in which compounds are purified and concentrated by chemical means, offer the same benefits as the whole food from which it is taken. What Drs Pauling and Sinclair both taught me is that cellular mechanisms select the natural isomers (compounds) it wants to incorporate into tissue. Eating purified extracts might not reproduce the benefits of eating fruits and vegetables that contain antioxidants and other agents found in the whole food.

You will be surprised by what we've learned about acai in the last decade that is now trickling into the scientific literature. As the senior author of two major papers on acai, I expect interest in acai by the research community will grow significantly. In just the last year, universities around the world have asked me to send them samples of the freeze-dried acai we've been studying. The resultant enthusiasm by the public once they hear more and more about this "super food" will stimulate purchasing products containing "acai." Approach these products with caution. Not all acai products are the same, and certainly many have far less antioxidant activity due to the way they have been processed, stored, shipped and repackaged into finished goods. In fact, as you will learn many acai powders and beverages have a fraction of the antioxidant activity they could have if processed to maintain the fruit's extraordinary antioxidant activity.

For this reason a particular freeze-dried powder of acai has generated considerable excitement following years of study in numerous laboratories. The findings of these laboratory studies will be a particular focus of this book, for they reveal the characteristics and attributes of a remarkable fruit previously appreciated by very few people in the world.

Chapter 1
What Is Açai Fruit?

Acai is a fruit that has two growing seasons borne by three related palm trees known to botanists as *Euterpe edulis*, *Euterpe oleracea*, and *Euterpe precatoria*. Palms fall within the family, Arecaceae (or Palmae, as some still call it), consisting of nearly 2700 species. Within the palm family are 200 genera (the plural for genus). These genera are organized into six subfamilies, and these subfamilies are in turn divided into tribes. *Euterpe precatoria*, *Euterpe edulis*, and *Euterpe oleracea*, are in the subfamily Arecoidaea, of the Arecea tribe.

Palms are monocots. They are very different from dicots, the trees most familiar to us, such as elms, maples, oaks, walnuts, pines, and firs; or fruit trees that bear apples, apricots, cherries, figs, nectarines, oranges, peaches, mangoes, and plums. The difference between monocots and dicots is important in understanding the ecological and nutritional issues that will be discussed in the chapters that follow.

If you cut off the top of a dicot tree, the tree does not die, but instead sends out new branches, one or more of which will try to replace the missing limb. By comparison, if you cut off the top of a monocot tree, no new lateral branches or limbs will form, and within a few weeks to months the tree will die.

Dicots tend to send roots deep into the earth, especially the taproot. By contrast, palms, a monocot, are only capable of significant lateral growth—basically, the roots spread out in every direction from the trunk not far below ground level; roots of some palms have been measured well over 100 feet away from the parent trunk. Another distinction is that dicots have root hairs designed to absorb nutrients and water, while palm roots do not have root hairs; rather, they grow just under ground level so they are close to extensive organic nutrient-rich areas of decomposing organic materials that filter nutrients to the root system.

Palms also have several methods of obtaining nutrients, which are different from dicots. One of the most important distinctions is that palms have what are known as *vascular bundles*. These bundles contain a highly developed network of cells that transfer carbohydrates manufactured in the leaves to other parts of the plant, while other bundles conduct water and dissolved minerals that have been absorbed by the roots to other parts of the palm.

The fruits (and seeds) of many palms are relatively large. A palm fruit consists of three layers: a thin outer surface called the epicarp; a thick fleshy fibrous section called the mesocarp (pulp); and a thick innermost layer called the endocarp. If you have ever eaten a husked coconut purchased in a supermarket, you are eating a palm fruit that has been cleaned down to the endocarp level (its thick innermost layer).

Palms are very difficult to grow via a technique called tissue culturing. This makes it difficult to grow palms wherever one wants. Tissue culturing consists of taking a piece of a plant (such as a stem tip, node, meristem, embryo, or even a seed) and placing it in a sterile, (usually gel-based) nutrient medium where it multiplies. The only species that have been successfully tissue cultured are two commercially important species: *Elaeis guineensis*, from which palm oil is derived, and *Phoenix dactylifera*, the palm that produces dates. All attempts to reproduce the acai palm outside of South America have failed, so it is apparent that the source of acai fruit will have to come from obtaining its fruit from palm trees growing in the wild, or those that have been cultivated on plantations in regions native to the wild palms.

E. oleracea and *E. edulis* are both found in South America. These are the only *Euterpe* palm species that grow the fruit known as "acai," although another member of Euterpe, *E. precatoria*, also has a fruit, but not of similar commercial value.

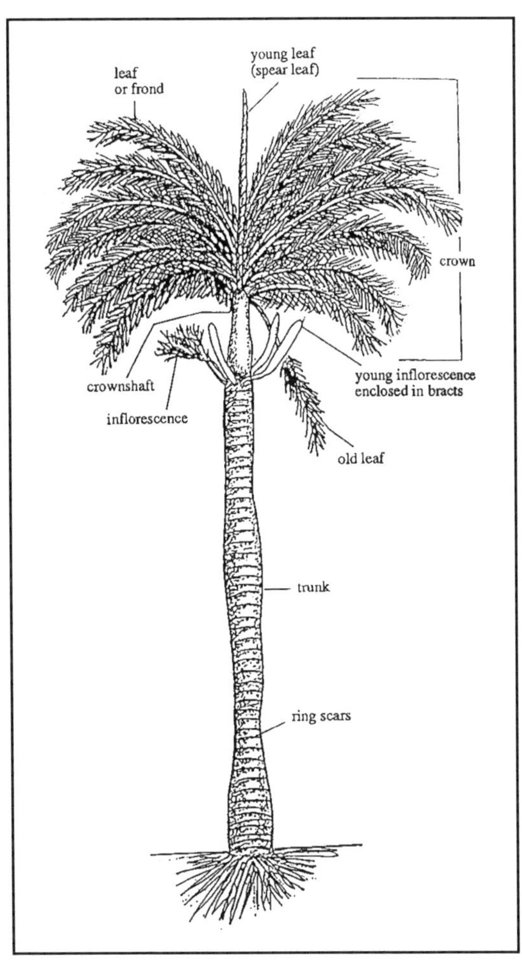

The tropical area known as Amazonia and its surrounding countries is the range and habitat for *E. edulis* and *E. oleracea*. These species can be found from the Atlantic coast of Brazil to forests on steep slopes farther inland, and from sea level to 3,300 feet (~1000 meters) in elevation. Just how far inland acai fruit can be found growing can be illustrated by the discovery of its use on the border of Brazil and Colombia, more than 2,500 miles from the Atlantic Ocean, among the Wanano Indians. In this region acai is called *wipi*. Among the Wanano Indians, wipi is a first-ranked fruit, very important to their hierarchical social system involving exchanges of different fruit. The Wanano distinguish "genus" and "species" levels of fruit, ranking them in relation to one another.

From this point on, we will refer to the acai palm interchangeably by its Latin name *Euterpe oleracea* (*E. oleracea*), since this is the palm tree that is the source of the frozen slurry and freeze-dried acai fruit pulp that has come into Europe, North America, and Japan in recent years, and is the subject of this book. But a few more comments about *E. oleracea* and *E. edulis* are in order before focusing just on the fruit of *E. oleracea*.

Euterpe translates from the Greek as "forest grace," owing to its elegant appearance—dropping leaflets that give the long pendulous fronds the appearance that rain had just fallen on them. Euterpe was also a Greek goddess of song and poetry, one of the nine muses of Greek mythology. For this reason, it is considered both by botanists and gardeners as one of the most attractive ornamental palms found in nature. Euterpe palms have been described as very graceful and easily recognizable by their slender gray stems, prominent crown shaft, and narrow pendulous leaflets.

E. oleracea is usually found growing along and near numerous tributaries that feed into the Amazon River system, and along the mighty river itself. By comparison, *E. edulis*, whose common names include juncara palm, palmito, and yayih, is usually found in the Atlantic coastal forests south of Sao Paulo.

Euterpe oleracea is a palm genus unique to the New World. Only 40 species of *Euterpe* are known. Three species, *E. precatoria*, *E. oleracea and E. edulis* provide edible fruit, but only the fruit of the latter species is referred to as "acai."

E. edulis is also the major source of heart-palms or what salad fans commonly call "heart-of-palm." *E. oleracea* can also provide heart-of-palm, but Brazilians prefer *E. edulis*, hence the reason groves of these palms have suffered the most. It is important to understand what has been happening in Brazil to understand the threat to sustainable sources of acai fruit.

Few people know that when they eat "heart-of-palm" in a salad or buy it in a supermarket to add to salads, they are actually eating the young top leaf, or spear found at the crown of the palm. To obtain the few feet of the heart of the palm to meet growing demand for this salad addition, the palm tree dies. There is no way to save the palm. This destruction can upset the ecology, as primates, birds and insects also favor it as a source of food and shelter.

The damage to the ecology of the Amazon due to world demand for heart-of-palm has even been the subject of a major article in *The Wall Street Journal* titled, "In Brazil, a Desperate Struggle is Waged Over a Salad Garnish." The *Journal* article reported that poachers illegally chop down 5,000 to 10,000 palm trees *a week*, just for the 12-to-16 inch (30 cm to 40 cm) section that might be found near the top of a 65 foot (19.8 meter) palm tree's trunk. Each poacher chops down an average of 50 trees a day, for $1 a trunk, according to Brazilian law enforcement authorities. Once the heart is removed, the tree dies. A palm tree that can be as much as 100 years old has just enough heart to fill two 14-oz. cans. When it reaches supermarket shelves in the United States, it will retail for about $3.99 per can.

To feed salad bars and salad connoisseurs worldwide, this poaching, and the resultant ultimate destruction of the palms, has been going on for so long that only 7% of the original Atlantic forest of Brazil is still standing. These forests are where the choicest heart-of-palm, the species *E. edulis*, comes from. With fewer and fewer palms, the poachers are beginning to encroach into other areas of Brazil, such as the famous Itatlaia National Park, southwest of Rio de Janeiro, visited by thousands of tourists and native Brazilians each year. As palm after palm is illegally killed for a few inches of a salad garnish, more and more of the national park's wildlife including animals, birds, insects and rodents, that are reliant upon the acai fruit for sustenance, suffer from the palm's destruction. Armed guards are starting to move the poachers out of these national parks, but unfortunately, they are now taking their illegal activity farther north into the Amazon, where the last large stands and groves of wild uncultivated *E. oleracea* palms grow.

What is particularly sad is that the heart-of-palm has no particular nutritional value beyond its fiber. This is not, however, the case with the fruit, which has been found to have significant nutritional value, as will be discussed later.

Recent interest in the value of the fruit has begun to help local inhabitants realize that cutting down these precious palm trees just for a few inches of the top core of the tree, is nowhere near as economically valuable as leaving the palm alone. Every palm tree produces an abundant crop of fruit twice a year. In just a few years, the value of the palm fruit itself far exceeds the value of removing the top core of the palm. Fortunately these palms do regenerate from seeds, but to replace what is destroyed takes decades, in that time much of the ecology will change and it may be too late to get it back to its original state.

The deforestation of the Amazon rain forest in 2004 was the second worst ever, according to the Brazilian government. Satellite photos show that ranchers, soybean farmers and loggers burned and cut down a near record 10,088 square miles of rain forest in one year. If this were to occur in the United States, it would be equivalent to leaving the entire states of Massachusetts, Hawaii or Vermont, totally bare of their forests. In Europe, it would be the equivalent of the entire country of Belgium, for comparison purposes, losing all of its trees in one year, and with them the wildlife that relies on those trees. At the pace deforestation is occurring in Brazil, by 2010, it will leave an American state equivalent in size to Oregon or Colorado or all of the states of New England, without trees. Imagine the environmental destruction this would cause once heavy rains occurred or fires raged out of control. Now think of what IS occurring in Brazil, where an average rainfall of 9 feet (108 inches) comes down annually, and it doesn't take much imagination to think of the massive amount of rich organic top soil that will be lost to the ocean forever.

Let's put this into an even clearer sense of the importance of these events to those who might believe we aren't affected by what is going on in Brazil.

The Amazon carries more water than any other river in the world. It gathers waters not only from Brazil, but also parts of Bolivia, Ecuador, Peru, Colombia, French Guiana, Suriname, Guyana and Venezuela. Forty percent of the water of South America drains through the Amazon River and its tributaries (Amazonia). Even more remarkable is the fact that 28 *billion* gallons of water flow into the Atlantic Ocean from the Amazon *every minute*. This represents one-fifth of the fresh water entering the oceans in the entire world. This immense discharge of water is so great that it dilutes the salinity of the ocean for more than 100 miles out to sea from the mouth of the Amazon.

The Amazon River is also so long and wide, that a boat can navigate it inland from the sea for over 2,300 miles. This watershed, which covers half of Brazil, is also home to the world's greatest biodiversity.

Within the lowlands of the Amazon, stretching from the Andes in the east to the Atlantic Ocean, also lays the largest rain forest in the world. Because its vegetation continuously recycles carbon dioxide into oxygen, it has been described by some scientists as the "lungs of our planet." Need to be convinced? Think of this: it supplies 20% of the earth's oxygen! Consider this extraordinary statistic the next time you take a breath.

As is becoming obvious to even the most skeptical reader, continued deforestation of the Amazon watershed can have catastrophic effects on the world's climate, especially as more and more fossil fuel is released into the atmosphere. And it is not going to get any better in the near future. Each year in China, the country is building the equivalent of five cities the size of Philadelphia. With those cities comes the need for motorized transportation, from trucks and buses, to personal automobiles. Consumers are purchasing 50,000 cars *each day* in China. This appetite for fossil fuel driven cars only adds more carbon into the atmosphere—the very atmosphere that relies on plants to convert that carbon dioxide to oxygen. Simply stated, as less and less of Amazonia has the biodiversity needed to absorb carbon dioxide and convert it into oxygen, the consequential impact on global warming is obvious. We are already seeing its effects in terms of climate changes being reported around the world; glaciers from the Himalayas to Alaska and the Alps to Andes mountains, are all receding. Once many of these glaciers disappear, how will these mountains fill the rivers and streams that hundreds of millions of humans rely on for drinking water and to grow crops?

Annually over nine feet of rain comes down on the Amazon, fifty percent of which returns to the atmosphere via the forest's foliage. Imagine how many countries in the world would lose significant amounts of rainfall needed to grow food if the amount of rainfall declines. As more and more countries, particularly in Africa, feel the effect of the Brazilian Amazon's destruction, what will they do for the water they need to feed their populations?

In addition, over 500 mammals, nearly 500 reptiles, and one fifth of the world's birds live in the Amazon. Biologists estimate that nearly 2.5 million insect species make their home there, while the number of botanical species is still unknown, but estimated to be in the tens of thousands, not counting the remarkable variety and number of fungi, mosses and lichens. Some biologists estimate that in one square kilometer (247 acres) of the Amazon basin, over 75,000 types of trees and 150,000 species of higher plants exist, equivalent to approximately 90,000 tons of living plants.

One fifth of the Amazon has already been deforested. So this problem is becoming critical. Scientists and environmentalists worldwide are doing everything they can to preserve the remaining Amazonian forest. Locked somewhere in its midst could be breakthrough botanicals capable of curing diseases. To date, 121 drugs have had their origin from this vast tropical forest, and many more life-saving botanicals are yet to be found. And this is where the story of acai fruit comes in, as it may hold riches as an anti-aging food that is unfolding right this minute as you read this book.

So where does the acai palm fruit come from?

Chapter 2
The Source of Açai fruit

In the Amazon River estuary of Brazil, locals call the palm tree *E. oleracea*, "acai." Hence, the origin of the name of the fruit, "acai." There are 18 synonyms for the fruit in several languages that refer to the acai palm; acai (Brazil), acal, acaizerio (Brazil), assai (Brazil), jicara, jucara (Brazil), manac (Trinidad), manaca, manaka (Suriname), naidi (Colombia), palmiteiro (Brazil), pinapalm, piria, pinot (French Guiana), prasara, wapoe, wasei, and wipi. However, "acai" is by far the most common reference to the fruit and palm. In areas where the palm tree grows in vast numbers around the Amazon River and its tributaries, in and around residences far from large cities and towns, every part of the palm is utilized by local inhabitants: roots, stems, the embryonic tissue at the 'growing tips' of the stems and roots (called the apical meristem), leaf sheaths (fronds), and the fruit. When made into a liquid beverage, the acai fruit is so much a part of the diet of thousands of Brazilians that it would compare to the popularity of orange juice for breakfast in North America.

But acai wasn't always that popular. There was a time when few people outside of the Amazon or Brazilian Atlantic Forest knew of this fruit or could get access to it unless they traveled to lowland areas around the Amazon River. More than 50 years ago, when travel in and out of the Amazon was difficult, and roads were unreliable and rail service limited, very little of the acai fruit made its way out of the Amazon to the country's large cities. The reason was simple—lack of refrigeration.

Without a way to keep the fruit refrigerated it quickly deteriorates, just as about every plant does in the tropics once it begins decaying. Without the enzymes found in plants that go into action when a plant or a plant part dies, the Amazon would turn into a giant biomass that would reach into the skies. Only by significantly cooling down this process of enzymatic decay can the acai fruit be preserved so that people hundreds and even thousands of miles away can consume it.

In the last two decades a reliable and cost-effective transportation infrastructure has been created that includes large refrigeration facilities built in cities like Belem at the mouth of the Amazon River. Here the fruit can be frozen into large blocks and shipped by truck to consumers throughout Brazil, including Rio de Janeiro and Sao Paolo. (In 2005, Sao Paolo, had 18 million inhabitants, double the number of people that lived there just 30 years ago). Demand for acai has surged in recent years, bringing with it the attention of nutritionists and health care practitioners, who have wondered what is responsible for its popularity beyond it being an abundant fruit found in Amazonia. Why hadn't fruits rich in nutrients like vitamin C found in camu-camu (*Myrciaria dubia*) or passion fruit (*Passiflora edulis*), become equally as popular?

But before going into why the acai fruit has become the fruit of choice in Brazil, where it is found in everything from ice cream to shampoos, understanding more about the fruit and its habitat will give you insight into why it has the prospect of becoming an important anti-aging food.

Chapter 3
Where Does Açai Grow?

The distribution and commercial sources of acai palm vary. The range and habitat of *E. oleracea* goes from the Pacific coast of Colombia and Ecuador, to coastal regions of Venezuela, Trinidad, the Guianas and Brazil. It is in the low lying and wet areas near tidal flats adjacent to the sea, and farther inland along riverines, that it is found in greatest abundance, particularly in Brazil's Amazonia.

The prime commercial source of acai fruit from *E. oleracea* comes from the area where several rivers converge within the Amazon estuary, emptying along the northeastern corner of Brazil into the Atlantic Ocean, between the states of Para to the south and Macapa to the north. Here the commercial hub of this region is defined by the city of Belem, the capital of the state of Para, located at the confluence of the rivers Guama and Acara. Near these two rivers, and away from Belem, lie a number of small and large islands. One of these, just 1.5 miles (2.5 kilometers) from Belem, is the island known as "Ilha das Oncas." Farther away is a much larger island called Marajo, some 24 miles (40 kilometers) northwest of Belem. The island of Marajo is the approximate size of Denmark. Several rivers surround the island, including the Amazon along its shores to the north and northwest. It is among these small and large islands at the mouth of the Amazon that large areas of floodplains and tropical forest are found rich with acai palms. In many areas near Belem, acai is one of the most abundant natural species found in the Amazon estuaries. One of the last surveys, done in 1972, estimated that the coverage of acai-dominated forests is conservatively around 10,000 square kilometers.

The management of acai is evident wherever one goes when traveling in this region, particularly along the channels and shorelines where dense stands of acai, called *terreiros* or home gardens, are found. Although acai dominates these home gardens, lemon, cacao and mango trees often grow as well. Acai fruit that exceeds what the family needs is sold to wholesalers. A secondary source of acai fruit comes from locations at a greater distance from Belem in either managed forests, called matos, or forests that have not been tampered with, but where abundant amounts of acai palm can be found. A tertiary source is cultivated plantations of acai palm. These tend to be near Manus and Belem and within easy transport to wholesalers. Some traditional households, while favoring fruit production, also sell heart-of-palm as a by-product.

The acai palm has a thin trunk, which is sometimes slightly curved. The fruits are round or egg-shaped (referred to as globose), approximately six-tenths of an inch (1.5 centimeter) in size (about the size of a marble), clustered into bunches, which can be harvested and brought to the ground to be separated from their stems. This stem, rich in fruit, is called an infructesence. The external color of the fruit is a rich dark purple, almost black when mature. The pulp is a deep red-purple color. Approximately 80 percent of the fruit is the seed, hence, only 20 percent of the fruit provides the pulp that can be made into a beverage or added to food. The best time to harvest the fruit is in the dryer months of July and December, when the fruit reach maturity.

Along the shores of these large islands, and along rivers that feed into the Amazon and its tributaries, water levels can rise nearly 12 feet during the seasonal flooding periods known as *varzea*. Along river banks, acai palm grow to heights of around 20 meters, which means someone has to climb up the trunk to remove the fruit bunch (infructesences) found just below the crown shaft near the top of the tree. New daughter palms that spring up near the parent plant can bear fruit that are only six to seven feet (2 meters) off the ground, making for relatively easier harvesting. Farther inland, in low-lying forests, acai palm trees can grow over 100 feet (30 meters) above the forest canopy, and live for over 100 years. Here harvesting becomes more challenging, as the fruit is much farther from the ground and requires skilled harvesters able to climb these tall palms to obtain the fruit. Nevertheless, these majestic palms farther away from riverines and populations centers are being illegally poached for heart-of-palm.

In one study of the uses of acai palm made in the 1980's, it was noticed that acai was frequently found "around the small and scattered dwellings which nestle between the surrounding flood-plain forest and river." The principle use of the acai fruit is for the production of a liquid beverage. When fresh, it is consumed like a cold soup, thick with pulp and eaten with a spoon, not drunk. It forms the major and basic part of the diet of many of the inhabitants of the region.

An investigation into the uses of the acai palm was funded by the U.S. National Academy of Sciences (NAS) and reported by the World Wildlife Fund (WWF) in the 1980's. The authors of this report observed that, "Those who consume [acai fruit] often appear strong and full of energy." Conversations with, and observations of individuals and families by the scientists showed "it to be loved and desired by the very young and the very old." Short periods without it appeared to result in a kind of withdrawal symptoms. When this happens, locals scramble up a fruit-filled acai palm, using a climbing belt called the *peconha*. Soon after eating some of the fruit they feel their cravings dissipate. There is even a saying in the region, reported by the study that, "when one is without acai one feels a lacking or emptiness in the stomach."

Acai forms such an important part of the diet, that up to two liters a day of it is consumed by individuals in the region. It is eaten during each meal including breakfast, lunch and dinner.

In more populated villages and towns, certain establishments sell it. Sometimes lines form, as people want to be sure they get the last of the day's supply of acai to consume or take home.

Acai fruit is not a product that is only consumed by the poor, as some have claimed. Rather it is found in the homes of all socioeconomic groups. In cooking, it is mixed with other foods in the area; including shrimp, fish, farina (manioc flour), biscuits, or combinations thereof and sometimes sweetened with sugar or other fruits. One can find acai on the menu at almost every hotel with a kitchen in large cities near the Amazon River estuaries, particularly when it is in season, or available.

There are many ways to prepare acai, but the most basic is to remove the mesocarp from the seed (the middle layer of the pericarp or fruit wall which is the fleshy and succulent part). It is then mashed up and combined with varying amounts of water to make as thick a liquid as desired.

Prices for the different grades and thicknesses vary throughout the year depending on availability. When supplies are low, due to seasonal variations in fruit production, acai must come from some distances up river where the fruit may still be maturing. Thus, price variations occur between peak periods of production and collection. Acai producers and middlemen also rank the quality of the fruit on a scale from 1 to 3, based on the pulp's thickness and freshness.

The most desirable variety of acai liquid is purple in color, called *acai preto*. There is also a yellow type called *acai branco*.

Besides acai's use as a subsistence food that most families rely on almost daily, many other products are made from acai. One example is a purple ice cream called *acai preto*, not to be confused with the yellow fruit variety, made from *acai branco* (the yellow variety). Other products include acai milk shake, mousse, acai chocolates and even acai cakes.

As mentioned earlier, the seeds constitute 80% of the fruit. Once removed from the mesocarp (pulp) and skin, these seeds are an important source of food for livestock, particularly pigs. In many homes the seeds are simply thrown into the pigpen. Another use for the seeds is as a source of organic soil to grow plants. The soil is formed after composting the seeds until it turns into a rich dark brown moist composition that can either be used for home vegetable gardens or sold as soil adamant. In large population centers, one finds large bins full of the seeds or organic soil produced from these seeds sold to city dwellers. Given how commonly acai fruit is consumed, excess seeds from commercial producers of the fruit liquid find a ready market. The seeds can also be used to grow new palms, as it only takes a few months in the moist climate of the region for the seeds to sprout and seedlings to form.

Even the stem branches that hold the fruit are used; for example, to make brooms. Once the fruit is removed from the infructescence skeleton (stem) it is also used as mulch around other commercially important plants, including the tree *Theobroma cacao*, the source of cacao beans, which every chocolate lover knows is the source of chocolate.

With the growing popularity of acai liquid and its by-products, there is a growing appreciation for the palm's value, not just as a commodity food item, but also as a source of a highly nutritious and phytonutrient-rich food source for people around the world.

As mentioned earlier, the harvesting of heart-of-palm sections means the imminent-death of the palm tree. Once the short section of the palm heart has been cut out of the top of the tree, it is taken to commercial facilities where these sections are cut into standardized lengths and put into a bath of water, salt and citric acid until canned. Once sealed, the cans are placed in steaming water to be sterilized before being labeled and shipped. Acai fruit by comparison, is collected over several months each year during two peak harvest seasons, without threatening the palm tree's survival.

Interestingly, the Brazilian government is well aware of the effect of poaching of palms for heart-of-palm. They have encouraged extensive plantation production of another palm, *Bactris gasipaes*, which can produce quality heart-of-palm. Nevertheless, as long as there is a market for heart-of-palm and poachers are willing to kill 50 palms a day for a mere dollar for that day's work, his practice will continue. However, if left unchallenged it will significantly affect the ecology. For example, the bird Cinereous Tinamon (*Cryturellus cinereus*) specializes in eating the acai fruit, as well as its leaves and hard shells. The same goes for the Barred Woodcreeper (*Dendrocolaptes certhia*), which is also partial to acai palms because it eats the insects which are drawn to the fruit. Loss of acai palms threatens these bird species.

In summary, the acai palm is a significant element in the diet of the people who inhabit the floodplains of the Amazon estuary. Conservation efforts favor the use of the fruit over the destruction of the palm to obtain short sections of heart-of-palm. Fortunately, palm trees are now being grown on plantations to allow for cultivated sources of heart-of-palm. Hopefully this will decrease illegal destruction of palms by poachers. The commercialization of heart-of-palm can co-exist, but only with careful thought to the effects of losing palm trees in this complex Amazonian estuarine ecosystem.

Chapter 4
Nutritional Value of Açai

Acai fruit is rich in nutrients. The first studies on the nutrient composition of acai fruit were reported between 1936 and 1948. More recent studies started appearing in 1961 and continue to the present. Early studies focused on the major vitamins and a few minerals, while latter studies reported on other macronutrients, minerals and trace elements, and the proximate composition of the fruit's lipids, carbohydrates and proteins. What was apparent, even a half century ago, was that the acai fruit pulp was a source for a range of vitamins, minerals, trace elements, macronutrients, in combination with enough calories to almost serve as a meal replacement. The food chemistry studies helped nutritionists appreciate why this food could sustain life for inhabitants relying on acai fruit as a important part of their diet. It also explained why those who consumed acai fruit were so healthy and reported that it gave them a sense of energy and endurance not experienced when consuming other fruits or vegetables.

However, the problem with many of the earlier studies was a lack of attention to information that other scientists needed to be able to replicate their findings. Often the published papers lacked sufficient methodological detail to allow the reader to understand how the data was generated. Additionally, these early analytical studies were published in either Portuguese or French, while the prevailing scientific languages around the earlier dates mentioned were English or German. Further, because the acai fruit could only be consumed in Brazil in regions close to where the acai palm grew, little interest existed in the nutritional value of the fruit since people outside of Brazil would never be able consume it due to lack of refrigeration and drying technologies.

However, with the introduction of commercial refrigeration in the Amazon, acai and other fruits from the Amazon began to appear in markets in non-Amazonian areas of Brazil, Peru and Venezuela. Rising consumption data on acai fruit was in direct proportion to its commercial availability outside of its native habitat.

By the 1990's university labs in Brazil were becoming more sophisticated in accurately measuring the amounts of specific nutrients in acai. The only problem was that when all of the published studies on acai were organized into a table, results reported by different labs were inconsistent. This was probably due to variations in the analytical methods and the equipment used by various laboratories. For example, calorimetric measurements of the number of kilocalories per 100 grams of fruit ranged from a high of 247 in 1977, to a low of 80 in 1948, and lower still, at 66.3, in 1996. So what number would most accurately represent the number of calories per gram or ounce to put on a food label? Another example is potassium, a very important electrolyte. In this case, the published data reported values as high as 1185 mg per 100 grams, to a low of 499 mg per 100 grams. Obviously, this is too great a variation to know what to put on a nutrition label.

By the late 1990's however, highly sophisticated and validated methods had been developed within the field of food chemistry to resolve these concerns. Also, methods of preservation became readily available, such as freeze drying that would produce a more consistent product. AIBMR Life Sciences (AIBMR), a research institute noted over the last quarter of a century for its work in nutraceuticals, located in Puyallup, Washington, decided to use the most modern analytical methods. These methods could be found in the international edition of official validated methods of analysis published by the American Organization of Analytical Chemists (AOAC) in the year 2000. By using validated methods labs worldwide could reproduce the results with the same reference standard material.

To conduct its research, AIBMR relied upon independent laboratories with considerable expertise in food chemistry using AOAC methods. No commercial interest sponsored this research; rather it was funded by AIBMR as one of its many basic research projects looking into the characteristics and chemistry of interesting food or ingredient products found in nature.

What particularly stimulated intensive research into acai fruit was a discovery by one of AIBMR's staff in the 1990's while doing a literature search on Brazilian fruits. He found a study published in 1945 concerning the nutritive value of acai fruit. In the report, the authors stated that,

> "*the interpretation of analytical data permits us to ascertain [acai] to be an essentially energetic food, with a caloric value higher than that of milk and with a content of lipids twice as high . . . a food of high caloric value [and] content of the minerals, calcium, phosphorous, and iron, suggests nutritional benefits.*"

Over the next few years, AIBMR was able to locate other studies, most of which were published in Portuguese, that reported finding additional nutrients, such as vitamin A, in the fruit. Since many of the methods used 20 to 50 years ago to determine nutrient content are archaic by today's methods of analysis, AIBMR decided to have acai's nutrient content determined using validated AOAC methods. These results, published by this author and his colleagues, are now available in peer reviewed scientific journals with full descriptions of each method used for each nutrient and analyte. The published results of AIBMR's analytical work, which this author has been privileged to commission and communicate, determined that this fruit had an impressive nutritional profile compared to fruits found around the world. To begin with, the freeze-dried acai fruit (OptiAcai™, K2A LLC, Provo, Utah) was found to have the following nutrients in appreciable amounts per gram of weight:

Vitamin A (as beta carotene)
Vitamin C (as ascorbate ion)
Vitamin E (as d-alpha tocopherol)
Vitamin D (as cholecalciferol)
Vitamin B-1 (as thiamin)
Vitamin B-2 (as riboflavin)
Vitamin B-3 (as niacin/niacinamide)
Vitamin B-6 (as pyridoxine)
Vitamin B-12 (as cyanocobalamin)
Pantothenic acid (as free anion)
Biotin
Folic Acid
Inositol

Calcium
Magnesium
Copper
Chromium
Zinc
Iron
Sodium
Manganese
Selenium
Boron
Potassium
Molybdenum
Iodine

The lead (Pb) level was extraordinarily low, at 22 parts per *billion*, a nearly undetectable level, using highly sophisticated analytical methods for the determination of heavy metals.

Acai fruit is an excellent source of vitamin A. Many of the carotenoids, such as beta-carotene, found in passion fruit have varying degrees of vitamin A activity, as an essential fat-soluble vitamin that is important in skin health, vision, growth and reproduction. Acai fruit also provides a significant source of the mineral potassium, an important electrolyte in aiding heart muscle contraction, acid-base balance, and the maintenance of healthy blood pressure. Hence, it can serve as an alternative to other foods known for their potassium level, such as the banana and orange. Beta-carotene possesses the greatest pro-vitamin A activity of the nearly 500 carotenoids identified to date, and is particularly beneficial in helping protect cells from the destructive damage free radicals can cause. Unless stopped, free radicals can lead to formation of pre-cancerous cells. Studies have shown that diets rich in carotenoids are associated with a reduced risk of breast, cervical, lung, skin and stomach cancer. This has not, however, been seen with beta-carotene supplements when taken by smokers, based on two studies showing no such benefit. Most probably, these negative outcomes are due to using only one carotenoid, rather than a mixture of carotenoids as would be found in a food like acai fruit. Increasing epidemiological evidence shows that regular consumption of mixed carotenoids may also be important in reducing the risk of cardiovascular disease and cataracts, owing to their antioxidant activity.

Freeze-dried acai fruit also was found to have a highly desirable amount of healthy fats, including plant derived monounsaturated and polyunsaturated fatty acids and some saturated fats, all three of which are derived from the diet and needed for many important and essential metabolic functions. More than 60 percent of the fruit was monounsaturated fatty acids, a large proportion of which was oleic acid. You don't need to be concerned with the quantity of fat in your diet, rather you need to be concerned with the type of fat. Saturated fat is not the enemy. Saturated fats, found mostly in butter and cheese for example, are not as dangerous as many believe, especially when consumed in proportion to a larger quantity of mono-unsaturated and polyunsaturated fats, as found naturally in acai fruit. Further, the cholesterol content was 1.25 percent of the fruit. However, due to the non-specificity of the assay used, this value most likely represents plant sterols (see Chapter 7). Cholesterol is almost never found in plants, but closely related sterols are ubiquitous. The sodium level was also very low, at 0.25 percent of the fruit.

In looking at the amino acid composition, freeze-dried acai fruit again surprised the chemists. Every essential and non-essential amino acid was found in the fruit, including:

Aspartic acid
Threonine
Serine
Glutamic acid
Glycine
Alanine
Valine
Methionine
Isoleucine
Leucine
Tyrosine
Phenylalanine
Lysine
Histidine
Arginine
Proline
Hydroxyproline
Cystine
Tryptophan

From a pure energy standpoint, acai fruit provided around 130 calories per normal beverage serving size (25 grams). Dietary fiber, an important part of any diet, was also identified in the freeze-dried fruit, at 44 grams per 100 grams. Sugars, which included fructose, lactose, sucrose, glucose and maltose, were only 1 gram per 100 grams of the product, which is good news for those watching their sugar intake.

The real breakthrough came when AIBMR took an interest in the outside color and pulp of acai fruit, not for its potential as a coloring agent, which had been studied by one research group in the 1990's, but in terms of its possible antioxidant activity.

Pursuing research on its antioxidant activity resulted in a major discovery, confirmed by a series of *in vitro* assays, and repeated a number of times on different samples of the freeze-dried fruit (OptiAcai™, K2A, Provo, Utah). To appreciate the significance of this finding, it is important to understand what free radicals are and how antioxidants work.

Chapter 5
The Importance of Antioxidants in the Diet

Public health officials are urging consumers to eat several portions of fruits and vegetables every day to obtain *antioxidants*. Unfortunately, most people have little knowledge of what antioxidants are or why they are important.

The reader may first have heard about antioxidants some years ago when mention was made of what is now well known *as The French Paradox*. The French have a diet relatively high in fat, as do people in other European countries and in America, but the French have a decreased incidence of heart disease. This was attributed to the average polyphenol content of white grapes, found to be approximately 4,000 milligrams per kilogram. Did this mean that one had to drink two or three glasses of wine everyday to obtain polyphenols in fruits? What about those who need to or want to abstain from drinking alcoholic beverages? Can they get antioxidants from other fruits with similar benefits?

What is an Antioxidant?

Vitamins C and E are two examples of antioxidants we find in our diet. These vitamins scavenge nasty free radicals that can cause cell damage and lead to disease and illness. Free radicals, often used by the immune system to kill viruses and bacteria, can wreak havoc in humans, unless quenched by free-radical scavengers called antioxidants. Think of free radicals as cattle that are loose and rampaging around fields of planted crops causing damage everywhere they go as they run wild. To prevent such damage, cowboys are hired to round up the stray cattle and make sure they stay in place and graze. Antioxidants act the same way. They basically capture free radicals before they can do more harm as they move through cells at incredible speeds, potentially damaging millions of healthy functioning cells or causing damage to their DNA that can result in mutated or abnormal cells. Many antioxidants work by terminating the cycle of free radical destruction. These chain-breaking free radical scavengers are referred to as primary antioxidants. There are other antioxidants, such as oxygen quenchers and synergists that remove oxygen from the auto-oxidation process, or avert them from catalyzing peroxides to aldehydes and ketones, respectively, but this is beyond the scope of this book.

Antioxidants can bind up free radicals very quickly if available, before a chain reaction of free radicals causes damage, but if antioxidants are not available, any damage done cannot be undone.

Another way of looking at free radicals is to think about the two-edged sword that oxygen provides us. On the one hand it gives us life, but on the other hand it can cause death. Hence, the reason we would never want to breathe pure oxygen for too long. Oxygen causes the body to age or basically rust. So think of free radicals formed as by-products of excessive oxygen as the same as rusting, and you get another way of viewing what excessive *oxygen free radicals* are doing to your health.

For the purposes of our discussion of antioxidant activity in acai fruit, it becomes necessary to introduce another term, *polyphenols*; commonly found in higher plants, such as fruit-bearing trees and shrubs. They serve as a diverse group of *polymeric* compounds containing multiple *phenolic* functions.

In *in vitro* (out of body) assays, vitamin E, a known antioxidant is used as a standard against which antioxidant activity of an ingredient or food can be measured. Polyphenols are classified according to their repeating monomeric building blocks. In the case of a fruit such as a grape, these monomers generally fall into two classes: flavonoids and non-flavonoids. The flavonoid polymers known as proanthocyanidins contain a specific type of flavonoid as monomers, called flavanols. The non-flavonoid polymers that are known as anthocyanins are composed of esters of the monomers.

What is also important is that polyphenolic compounds have repeatedly been demonstrated to inhibit lipoxygenase and cyclooxygenase enzymes and lipid peroxidation *in vitro*, and to scavenge hydroxyl, peroxyl and superoxide radicals, free radicals. What this means is that polyphenolics may play an important role in preventing cardiovascular diseases such as arteriosclerosis and atherosclerosis, disease processes which if allowed to progress, can result in heart damage, heart failure and stroke.

Several studies have found both an increased antioxidant capacity of human blood plasma following ingestion of polyphenols, followed by a decrease in the level of LDL-cholesterol oxidation. How often do you read or hear someone say, reduce your LDL-cholesterol and raise your HDL cholesterol? Well, what scientists have learned in recent years is, that polyphenols decrease harmful LDL-cholesterol that contributes to the build-up of plaque in arteries that eventually leads to inflammation and a catastrophic blockage of an artery.

Let's get a bit more technical again to appreciate the profound discovery of freeze-dried acai fruit (OptiAcai™) antioxidant activity made by AIBMR.

A number of studies have established a relationship between the structure of different flavonoids and their relative efficiencies as antioxidants, which are also referred to as reducing agents. Basically, reducing agents can donate an electron to a free radical, thereby stabilizing and inactivating the damaging radical, a process called hydroxylation. In this process, the polyphenolic reducing agent becomes an aroxyl radical, which is considerably more stable than the free radical that it has reduced. When this happens, the damaging oxidative chain reaction is stopped. But this process, repeated too often, can exhaust the hydroxylation that needs to continue due to a diminishing number of hydrogen atoms. This is where vitamin C comes in. Vitamin C works with polyphenolics by regenerating the hydrogen atoms that are lost during this reducing activity. Hence, the presence of vitamin C-rich fruits, such as acerola and passion fruit, found in South America might be worth combining together in a beverage to ensure that hydroxylation can continue when needed. Fortunately acai fruit contains vitamin C, as pointed out earlier, but there is another fruit from the same area of the world that acai comes from that deserves mention, passion fruit.

Passion fruit (*Passiflora edulis*), commonly called *Maracuya* in South America, is a purple fruit native to southern Brazil, Paraguay and northern Argentina. It was named by the Spanish missionaries arriving in the New World who saw the passion (or suffering) of Christ represented in its flowers. Passion fruit is the richest source of vitamin C of any fruit found in nature. One glass of passion fruit juice provides about 50% of the dietary intake for adult men and 60% for women for vitamin C. For this reason it would require very little of the fruit to aid in the work that polyphenols are performing to ensure that hydrogen atoms are replenished. This would continue free radical scavenging that might be needed to break free radical chain reactions that might suddenly occur with all their destruction of healthy cells.

Another factor that influences the antioxidant capacity of a flavonoid is the degree of hydroxylation on the 'B' ring. Without going into the chemistry of this, just know that the degree of antioxidant capacity with increasing hydroxylation is continued with compounds called *proanthocyanidins*, also found in the acai fruit. This trend of increasing antioxidant capacity with increasing degrees of hydroxylation is continued with the multiple-hydroxylated oligomeric proanthocyanidins. This observation agrees well with studies that have indicated, for example, that the soluble condensed tannins of red wine are the major contributors to its total antioxidant capacity.

When we eat fruits or vegetables, we ingest a complex mixture of phenolic compounds. Epidemiological evidence suggests that maximum antioxidant benefit results from the balance and concentration of polyphenols and other antioxidants found in foods that represent a spectrum of antioxidant-rich foods.

One way of measuring the antioxidant capacity of a food is the ORAC assay. As mentioned in the introduction, the oxygen radical absorption capacity (ORAC) assay looks at how much a particular food inhibits free radical activity. There are several different ORAC assays, each of which had been conducted on freeze-dried acai.

A scientist at the National Institutes of Aging developed the ORAC assay in 1992. In 1996, this scientist joined the United States Department of Agriculture (USDA) Human Nutrition Research Center on Aging in Boston to develop a semi-automated method for the ORAC assay. This assay was declared to be one of the greatest technological developments ever made by the USDA in over 120 years. Since then, the ORAC assay has been repeatedly validated as a reliable method for antioxidant capacity determination and extensively utilized in the field of antioxidant and oxidative stress research involving food and animals, including humans.

The concept of ORAC is based on a hydrogen atom transfer reaction mechanism relevant to what goes on in human biology. In the ORAC assay, Trolox, a water-soluble analogue of vitamin E is used as a control-everything is compared against this vitamin E analogue. Results are expressed as an ORAC value in micromoles of Trolox equivalents (TE) per gram. (One gram is equal to 0.03527 ounces, hence 100 grams would be equivalent to approximately 3.5 ounces.) The USDA Agricultural Research Service (USDA/ARS) facility at the University of Arkansas, and the leading commercial laboratory that performs ORAC assays, Brunswick Laboratories (Wareham, MA), have determined that there is a broad range of antioxidant activity in foods Americans eat, from a low of 2 TE/gram for tomato to the highest recorded for any food we eat, 95 TE/gram for cranberries. This range was determined after USDA/ARS performed hundreds of assays on every food customarily consumed by Americans that might have antioxidant activity, including changes in antioxidant activity of those foods that might occur during different seasons of the year. So keep that highest number in mind—95, to appreciate how high the ORAC value is for freeze-dried acai fruit.

Commercial labs occasionally report higher ORAC values for some foods because they only receive one or two samples from the submitter. For this reason the USDA/ARS data relies on numerous samples studied taking into account seasonal variation of antioxidant levels in foods.

One of the other things that makes the acai fruit interesting, beyond its nutritional value and history of traditional use, is its pigmentation. Anthocyanins, a group of natural phenolic compounds, are plant pigments that are widely distributed in nature. They basically give fruits, berries and vegetables their colors. Hence, colorful foods are major sources of anthocyanins in the diet. Recently, scientists have given considerable attention to their possible health benefits in preventing chronic and degenerative diseases, including heart disease and cancer. Recent evidence is attributing these benefits to their antioxidant capacity.

Dietary antioxidants, including vitamins C and E, and particularly polyphenolic compounds, are thought to be important nutrients in the prevention of oxidative stress. Hence, regular consumption of antioxidants in the diet is believed to be a contributing factor in decreasing the risk of diseases associated with aging and conditions associated with oxidative stress.

Prior to ending this chapter, a caveat is necessary before leaving the subject of *in vitro* antioxidant assay testing. It is good to remember that *in vitro* results may or may not be directly equivalent to "real-life" situations *in vivo* (in the body). To make progress in extrapolating *in vitro* results to their applications *in vivo*, scientists are rapidly developing and testing for bioactivity in cell culture systems. This is a rapidly emerging tool in research, especially as it relates to the effect of antioxidants on specific cell types. For example, a study by the University of Florida published in 2006 found that acai's polyphenolics have an antiproliferative effect and ability to cause cell death of HL-60 human leukemia cells. Does that mean it will prevent or treat leukemia? We just don't know at this time. But seeing such an effect might justify conducting human clinical trials.

Additional progress has been made by the development of oxidative stress panels. These panels allow one to have his or her blood or urine checked for baseline antioxidant activity and then compare the response the same variables following ingestion of antioxidant foods over time. Some examples of such panels are the plasma ORAC, plasma T-Bars, urine total peroxides, DNA damage markers and protein damage markers.

Antioxidants from dietary sources interact with the free radicals in the body to inhibit oxidative damage to cell membranes and DNA. These dietary antioxidants do not necessarily alter the antioxidant level in the body, but they may decrease the oxidative stress level. That's an important point to understand. Oxidative stress levels are determined by the quantity of oxidized products of lipids, proteins and DNA. In general, the higher the ORAC value of an antioxidant-rich food, the lower the level of oxidative stress will be measured, provided that the given antioxidant possesses relatively high bioavailability.

Why this is important to know is that the etiology (cause or origin) of many of the major degenerative diseases, such as cancer, atherosclerosis, diabetes, etc, suggests they are initiated by the reaction of free radicals with lipids, proteins and DNA. More important, there is growing evidence that the onset and incidence of these diseases may be retarded by regular intake of fruits and vegetables.

Further, it is recognized that the activity of an antioxidant compound may be influenced by numerous factors, such as lifestyle (e.g. alcohol intake, smoking, occupational toxins, etc), dietary factors, and the presence of chronic infections or diseases, as modified by the enzymatic and microbial environment of the individual's human digestive system. What this means it that it may be possible that the metabolites produced by bacteria in the gut from polyphenolic compounds and antioxidant vitamins may be as important or even more important than the parent compounds.

There is emerging evidence that in some cases these metabolites themselves serve as antioxidants *in vivo*. If proven true, then the bottom line is to supply the body with polyphenolic compounds and antioxidant vitamins on a regular basis, but within the range of physiologic requirements needed by the body, and then let the body and its digestive system and its bacterial hosts in the gut determine what is needed. This may also suggest that consumption of blends of different fruit juices with acai fruit could impart unique functional attributes that could be an effective strategy for the development of a diet-based approach toward the prevention and/or management of oxidative stress linked diseases.

Chapter 6
The Highest Antioxidant Capacity of Any Fruit or Vegetable

In the last chapter it was pointed out that free radicals are the lead agents of interest in research related to antioxidants and oxidative stress. Free radicals are reactive species (called oxidants) that can have adverse effects on normal physiological function, which we refer to as oxidative stress. The role of antioxidants then is to interact with excessive free radical activity and mop or quench them up so they are rendered harmless. One way to determine if a food, such as the acai fruit, has this potential is to have assays performed *in vitro* to measure their activity against radical and non-radical oxidants: the peroxyl, superoxide, and hydroxyl radicals, peroxynitrite, and singlet oxygen, respectively. Peroxynitrite, for example, is a strong oxidant, which can damage proteins, DNA and other cellular structures, when produced by the immune system as part of its natural cellular defense system. In other words, free radicals are not all bad, since they play a role in killing pathogens that enter our body or destroy cancer cells. There is a problem when their damaging effects against pathogens or cancer cells aren't managed. When that occurs, it can cause oxidative damage to healthy cells as a by-product of their function in keeping us healthy.

Oxidative stress is the adverse effect of oxidants on physiological function. This stress has been implicated in the progression of aging and disease. There is mounting evidence from studies worldwide that this stress can be reduced by antioxidants.

In the previous chapter it was mentioned that the USDA has tested all of the fruits and vegetables consumed in the United States for their antioxidant activity via the ORAC assay. The USDA reports that the highest average ORAC of any of the foods they tested was for cranberries, which came out with a Total (hydrophilic and lipophilic) ORAC score of 95.

You can imagine my response when we tested a sample of freeze-dried acai fruit pulp (OptiAcai™) provided to us years ago using the same methods to determine its antioxidant activity as used by the USDA. The Total ORAC value was *1027*, basically and literally off the charts. Essentially, this made freeze-dried acai fruit pulp the star among well-known antioxidants, such as blueberries, grapes, red wine, green tea, cranberries, blackberries, pomegranates, orange juice, and any of the exotic beverages of fruits from Asia, such as mangosteen *(Garcinia mangostana)*, noni *(Morinda citrifolia)*, or wolfberry *(Lycium chinensis)*. Could the results be a fluke?

To ensure that the result wasn't spurious, we had numerous samples tested during different seasons of fruiting and over several years. Still the outcome showed it to have the highest antioxidant activity based on the ORAC assay of any food in the American diet. We also tested other drying methods to preserve acai and bring it out of the Amazon to markets such as the United States, including spray drying and thin film drying, but neither of these approached the same high value seen with freeze drying. In fact, they proved to be significantly lower, especially samples that were spray-dried and then shipped across the ocean as frozen pulp and thereafter reprocessed. Why is freeze drying superior to other drying methods?

Walter S. Pebley, a professional engineer and authority on freeze drying, and James S. Baglien, a physiologist, can provide an explanation.

> "Freeze drying is a process in which water is removed as vapor directly from ice, without passing through the liquid state. This process is called sublimation, and requires reduced pressure to occur. All other drying methods use evaporation; that is, water is removed as vapor from liquid water with heated air. Freeze dried acai does not require heat in the sublimation process."

Freeze drying of acai fruit is effective in permitting the fruit to retain its original characteristics of color, form, taste, size and nutrient content. There are several reasons for this. First, freezing slows or stops most chemical reactions, especially important when dealing with a tropical fruit that, once removed from its parent host, is programmed to rapidly decay. Second, the process occurs under a vacuum in the absence of oxygen. This prevents oxidative reactions to occur. Third, it can be performed at very low temperatures—lower than by any other drying method. At these low temperatures, enzymatic and bacterial breakdown cannot occur. Further, chemical changes that might occur are minimized.

Unlike acai pulp that is exported while still containing its moisture content (which basically means a LOT of water is being shipped), once the fruit is freeze-dried, further cold storage is not required.

Other benefits of freeze-drying are that it reconstitutes to its original state when placed in water; it remains shelf stable at room temperature, the weight of the product is reduced by 70 to 90 percent, and with no change in volume—making it lightweight and easy to handle. Low water content of freeze-dried acai virtually eliminates microbiological concerns (which have been supported by shelf-life studies).

Another approach might have been to have the fruit pulp exported as a puree. However, a puree should be pasteurized, which can change some of its characteristics, such as color and taste. It would require sugar or some other additive to the product. Since a puree must be heated, certain nutrient levels might significantly decline, such as the heat labile vitamins; and the color and taste of the fruit altered.

Understanding the advantages of freeze-drying explains why astronauts out in space with no fresh food to consume can survive for months eating a diet of freeze-dried foods. The advantage we have on earth is that the freeze-dried powder can be added to water to rehydrate it and then sealed until opened by the consumer.

According to data published in 2004 and 2005 by the USDA in *the Journal of Agricultural and Food Chemistry*, one can compare acai's Total ORAC value to common fruits and vegetables on a gram to gram basis as shown in Tables 1 and 2.

Table 1

Comparison of ORAC Values (Antioxidant Activity) in Fresh Fruit

Fresh or Raw Fruit	*Total ORAC (micromoles TE/g)*
Acai fruit (freeze-dried OptiAcai)	*1027*
Acai fruit (fresh)	*185*
Cranberry	95
Blueberry (low bush)	93
Plums (black)	73
Plums	62
Blueberry (cultivated)	62
Blackberry	53
Raspberry	49
Apple, Red Delicious (with peel)	43
Acai fruit, frozen	40*
Apple, Granny Smith	39
Strawberry	36
Cherries (sweet)	34
Apple, Red Delicious (no peel)	29
Apple, Gala	28
Apple, Golden Delicious (with peel)	27
Apple, Fuji	26
Apple, Golden Delicious (no peel)	22
Applesauce	20
Avocado (Haas)	19
Pears (green cultivars)	19
Pear (Red Anjou)	18
Orange (Navel)	18
Peaches	18
Tangerines	16
Grapefruit (red)	16
Apricot	13
Grapes (red)	13
Grapes (green)	11
Mango	10
Kiwifruit	9
Bananas	9
Pineapples	8
Nectarines	8
Peaches, canned in heavy syrup	4
Cantaloupe	3
Honeydew melons	2
Watermelon	1

*Lab analysis of hydrophilic ORAC value only (Brunswick Labs, 2005), Schauss, AG et al. *Federation of Societies Experimental Biology Journal*, 2006c.)

(Source: Wu, X et al. *Journal of Food Composition and Analysis*, 2004; Wu, X et al. *Journal of Agricultural and Food Chemistry*, 2004; Schauss AG et al. Journal of Agricultural and Food Chemistry, 2006a; Schauss AG et al. Journal of Agricultural and Food Chemistry, 2006b; Schauss, AG et al. *Federation of Societies Experimental Biology Journal*, 2006c.)

Table 2

Comparison of ORAC Values (Antioxidant Activity) in Fresh, Raw And/or Cooked Vegetables

Fresh, Raw or Cooked Vegetables	*Total ORAC (micromoles TE/g)*
Acai fruit *(Freeze-dried OptiAcai)*	*1027*
Acai fruit (fresh)	*185*
Acai spray-dried powders	*55-155*
Artichoke	94
Peas (black eye)	43
Butterhead lettuce	33
Cabbage (red)	31
Broccoli (raab)	30
Asparagus	30
Beets	28
Spinach	26
Eggplant	25
Broccoli	16
Potato, Russet, cooked	16
Potato, red, cooked	13
Carrot	12
Green leaf lettuce	12
Red lead lettuce	12
Onions, yellow and red	11
Potato, white, cooked	11
Radishes	10
Salsa	10
Peppers, red sweet	9
Romaine lettuce	9
Sweet potato, cooked	8
Cauliflower	6
Celery	6
Green Peas, frozen	6
Ketchup	6
Peppers, Green Sweet (Bell Peppers)	6
Iceberg Lettuce	6
Tomato Juice	6
V8 Vegetable Juice	6
Corn, frozen	5
Pumpkin, raw	5
Corn, canned	4
Green Peas, canned	4
Snap Beans, canned or raw	3
Tomato, raw	3
Lima Beans, canned	2
Cucumber, with and without peel	1

(Source: Wu, X et al. *Journal of Food Composition and Analysis*, 2004; Wu, X et al. *Journal of Agricultural and Food Chemistry*, 2004; Schauss AG et al. Journal of Agricultural and Food Chemistry, 2006a; Schauss AG et al. Journal of Agricultural and Food Chemistry, 2006b; Schauss, AG et al. *Federation of Societies Experimental Biology Journal*, 2006c.)

However, Tables 1 and 2 would not be a fair comparison between freeze-dried acai fruit and other common fruits and vegetables because there is a difference in the water content between fresh fruit and dried fruit. So a more accurate comparison would be to adjust for moisture content of each food sample assayed. Brunswick Laboratories (Wareham, MA), a leading ORAC assay lab that has published its validated analytical method, provided the data for common foods and freeze-dried acai as shown in Table 3. These results have been adjusted for moisture content on a gram-to-gram basis.

Table 3

Comparison of ORAC Values (Antioxidant Activity)

in Dried Fruits and Vegetables

Dried Fruits & Vegetables	*ORAC value (micromoles of TE/g)*
Acai (freeze-dried OptiAcai)	1027
Wild black raspberry	340
Wild blueberry	260
Elderberry	240
Wolfberry	220
Red raspberry	210
Green pepper	160
Spinach	150
Beans, dry, mature (small red)	149
Beans, dry, mature (red kidney)	144
Beans, dry, mature (pinto)	124
Hawthorn	130
Broccoli	130
Cranberry	125
Beets	120
Cherry	100
Red pepper	90
Prunes	86
Beans, dry, mature (black)	80
Green beans	70
Acai spray-dried powder	*60**
Tomato	60
Carrot	50
Dates, Deglet Noor	39
Figs	34
Raisins	30
Dates, Medjool	24

*Lab analysis of hydrophilic ORAC value only (Brunswick Labs, 2005), Schauss, AG et al. *Federation of Societies Experimental Biology Journal*, 2006c.)

(Source: Wu, X et al. *Journal of Food Composition and Analysis*, 2004; Wu, X et al. *Journal of Agricultural and Food Chemistry*, 2004; Schauss AG et al. Journal of Agricultural and Food Chemistry, 2006a; Schauss AG et al. Journal of Agricultural and Food Chemistry, 2006b; Schauss, AG et al. *Federation of Societies Experimental Biology Journal*, 2006c.)

In Table 3, dehydrated fruits and vegetables are compared to freeze-dried acai fruit. In this case all of the foods tested have almost all of the moisture removed before being assayed. Again, the results are similar to those seen in tables 1 and 2, in that freeze-dried acai fruit was superior in total antioxidant capacity to other foods even when compared on a head-to-head, direct basis.

As shown in Table 1, "Acai, fresh" fruit, only had a Total ORAC of 185, against a sample provided by K2A that has the acai freeze dried in Brazil, which had a value of 1,027. Why such a huge difference? The fresh sample was harvested in Brazil and flown directly into the USA and sent to the lab to be assayed within three days of being harvested from the palm tree. This illustrates how quickly the level of antioxidant activity declines, and the reason so much research on acai, as reported in 2006 in two major papers on its composition and bioactivities, was performed on the freeze-dried powder. Acai may be a "Super Food", as described by a noted physician at Harvard University in his book, *The Perricone Promise*, but is only super when the source is truly fresh acai, as can be consumed in the Amazon, or when preserved via freeze drying.

In summary, no matter how one tries to compare different foods to acai fruit or freeze-dried acai fruit pulp, the freeze-dried pulp is superior in oxygen radical absorption scavenging capacity (ORAC) *in vitro* to all other fruits and vegetables, when controlled for moisture content.

But there is another finding that is equally as important as acai's remarkably high ORAC value compared to other foods. In 2006, it was reported that "freeze-dried Acai [OptiAcai™] fruit pulp/skin powder has been shown extremely powerful in its antioxidant properties against superoxide (($O_2^{\bullet -}$) by the SOD assay." As pointed out by the authors, "superoxide is believed to the cause of other radical oxygen species (ROS) formation, such as hydrogen peroxide, peroxynitrite and hydroxyl radicals. Therefore, superoxide scavenging capacity in the human body is the first line of defense against oxidative stress." Further, they pointed out that, "superoxide scavenging capacity in blood is considered very important in maintaining antioxidant status."

It turns out that freeze-dried acai has a superoxide scavenging capacity of 1614 units/gram, meaning the freeze-dried powder has extremely high scavenging capacity to superoxide, by far the highest of any fruit or vegetable tested. To get an appreciation of how high this is, consider that the next highest superoxide scavenging capacity from any natural source is wheat sprout juice, ranging from 160 to 500 units/gram for different samples tested.

As a scientist, I find it remarkable that Dr. Nathan Perricone considered this fruit among his top "Super Food" selections in the book, "The Perricone Promise", well before its superior peroxyl radical and superoxide scavenging capacity had been reported in the scientific literature, as his book predates the publication of these discoveries.

In his follow-up book, *The Perricone Weight-loss Diet*, published in 2005, Dr. Perricone states:

"Because of the excellent fatty acid, amino acid, and anti-inflammatory profile, it deserves star billing ... One of the qualities I love about acai is that it provides us quality protein, healthy fat, and powerful antioxidants all in one amazing berry." (pp. 58-59)

His mention of acai containing "healthy fat", relates to it being rich in monounsaturated oleic acid, the primary fatty acid found in olive oil. Oleic acid helps fish oils penetrate the cell membrane, providing them suppleness and flexibility. In Dr. Perricone's opinion this allows, "all hormones, neurotransmitters, and insulin receptors to function more efficiently; critically important to maintain homeostasis, that is, keeping the body working as it should because all of its systems are in balance."[p.59] Only when this happens does he believe it can contribute to weight loss and reduce the likelihood of gaining unwanted weight.

He then goes on to explain why he selected acai for his book on weight-loss.

"Acai is good for weight loss because it contains cyanidin, a highly antioxidant phytochemical compound."

He bases this claim on Japanese research that had discovered cyanins might work by reducing fat absorption and "draining body fat."[p.59]

And yet there is still more data that was reported in 2006 on acai's antioxidant activity. Besides acai's ability to show superior free radical scavenging activity *in vitro* against the peroxyl radical and superoxide compared to any other food, studies have been carried out using two other assays, the HORAC and the NORAC, to further elucidate its antioxidant activities.

The most common radical oxygen species our body produces *in vivo* are superoxide ($O_2^{\bullet-}$), hydroxyl radical ($OH^{\bullet}$), peroxyl radical ($RO_2^{\bullet}$), nitric oxide ($^{\bullet}NO$) and peroxynitrite ($ONOO^{-}$). These free radical species have been associated with many degenerative and chronic diseases, and overall aging. By performing two additional antioxidant assays, we get a more complete picture of acai's free radical scavenging capacity. Hence, the two additional assay results of interest reported in 2006 include the HORAC, which measures the hydroxyl radical averting capacity, and the NORAC which determines the peroxynitrite radical averting capacity.

Hydroxyl radicals are short lived but the most damaging of radicals. It is formed by interaction of copper or iron. This explains why when men get older, and women are post-menopausal, iron intake from the diet should be limited to what is required to maintain health. Iron is required as a component of the oxygen carrying proteins (myoglobin and hemoglobin) that transport oxygen from the lungs to our tissues. Hence, iron, an essential trace element, is in contact with oxygen.

Peroxynitrite is another oxidant which can cause damage to proteins, cells, and DNA. It occurs when superoxide and nitric oxide react or other compounds find each other in the body. Unfortunately, some of the chemical reactions escape control, and when they do, free radicals induced by these reactions appear that can cause peroxynitrite-related damage to the body.

Both assays found that freeze-fried acai also had antioxidant capacity against the hydroxyl radical and peroxynitrite.

If you feel freeze-dried acai between your fingers, you will note it has an oily consistency, suggesting that it may contain large amounts of what are called "lipophilic" compounds capable of combing with or dissolving lipids (fats). As in the case of so much research on acai, in 2006 it was reported that the freeze-dried acai lipophilic ORAC is the highest of any berry samples tested to date. This means it has the potential, if clinically demonstrated *in vivo*, to be a dietary food source with potential free radical scavenging activity useful in reducing lipid oxidation. For nearly twenty years it has been important to learn which compounds in foods inhibit oxidation of various biological lipid systems, implicated in the initiation and development of atherosclerosis. Whether acai will be able to do so needs to be demonstrated, but that its lipophilic antioxidant activity exceeds that of any other berry may just encourage such research.

That brings us to one of the most puzzling findings about acai. When freeze-dried acai was found to have an extraordinarily high Total ORAC capacity, it was assumed this meant it had the highest content of the compounds that can be attributed to its antioxidant activity as a food, namely, anthocyanins, proanthocyanidins and other polyphenolic compounds. But to the scientists at USDA that measured the levels of these compounds, the freeze-dried acai powder had much lower levels than found in blueberries or other berries with elevated Total ORAC values. Then to make it even more puzzling, the following was reported, again in 2006:

> "To make things even more confusing, the total phenolics in Acai was found to be only 13.9 mg/g GAE. In a recent paper, the ratio between hydrophilic $ORAC_{FL}$ and total phenolics was found to vary dramatically from less than two to more than 100 for different groups of foods (*14*). For most fruits and vegetables, this ratio is about 10. However, the ratio in Acai is 50, five times greater than that found for any other fruit. This "unusual" ratio raises questions whether or not Acai contain much stronger antioxidants than found in other berries on an equal weight basis."

Work is already underway to determine why acai has antioxidants so much more powerful than any other fruit. But some answers related to this question can be provided.

Why Does Açai Have So Much Antioxidant Activity?

Given that many fruits and vegetables are rich in polyphenols, anthocyanins (which give the food its color), and tannins, why is it that acai fruit's ORAC assay would be so much higher than any other common food? For years I kept wondering what the answer is. Finally, I went back to basics as to why plants use up the energy to produce antioxidant compounds to begin with. The answer was obvious: to cope with oxidative stress. So what kind of stresses does an acai palm go through that would give it such an unusually high antioxidant capacity? If you look at where vast amounts of acai palm grow one would note that the plant is growing right near the equator where the sun is intense year round.

I will never forget my first experience some years ago when I was in the state of Kalimantan in Indonesia standing literally on the imaginary line that is known as the equator. By 11 AM I could feel my skin almost burn in minutes from the intense ultraviolet (UV) radiation on the particularly (rare) clear day I was doing some research there.

The acai palm, which grows densely near the equator in Brazil, only needs shade during its early years of development through its juvenile stage. Once it starts getting tall, it can withstand more and more UV radiation. As it reaches its maximum height of 65 to 100 feet (20 to 30 meters), it becomes a member of the tropical forest's canopy. This is particularly true in the low lands near rivers and their tributaries and along coastal swamps.

Swamps? What happens in swamps but seasonal flooding? If you put a tropical food crop like corn under water for more than a few days, it will die. It is a condition called anoxia, caused by a lack of oxygen. Clearly a stress condition, which if prolonged, can easily kill a plant. Unlike most plants that cannot live in a state of anoxia for very long, the acai palm can withstand weeks, even months of flooding. This is possible because of oxygen diffusion that takes place from its leaves into the roots where aerobic respiration can occur at the same time that anaerobic metabolism occurs.

In the acai palm, energy in the form of adenosine triphosphate (ATP) continues to be synthesized in cells in the absence of oxygen. Rice can do this too. That explains why it does so well in paddies filled with water. So this is not an ordinary palm, but one that has evolved over time to cope with all kinds of severe climatic and geologic stresses, particularly flooding. Not surprising when one considers that it rains almost every day in the Amazon.

How each stressor directly causes an increase in the production of antioxidant compounds remains to be learned. But it helps to understand why two plants, such as an eggplant, which also has a very dark skin full of anthocyanins, with low antioxidant absorbance capacity, and acai fruit; with extraordinarily high antioxidant absorbance capacity, would achieve such different ORAC scores.

Which Antioxidants Does Açai Have?

What antioxidant compounds are there in acai palm fruit? We have come close to fully characterizing (analyzing and determining) the composition of this fruit. Using highly sophisticated analytical methods involving mass spectroscopy, it has been determined that the freeze-dried acai fruit powder contains a number of anthocyanins, including cyanidin-3-glucoside and cyanidin-3-glucoside-coumarate, in addition to the following phenolic compounds: protocatechic acid, catechin and epi-catechin (yes, the same compounds found in green tea, chocolate, grapes, berries, and apples), eriodictyol-7-glucoside, luteolin-4-glucoside, isoquercitin, quercitin-3-arabinoside, eriodictyol (found in citrus fruits), luteolin, chrysoeriol, eupatorin, and kaempferol (found in onions, scallions, kale, broccoli, apples, berries and tea).

Chapter 7
Benefits of Antioxidants

Açai Safety

Before discussing the benefits of acai fruit pulp, the question might be asked—is it safe to eat? My research found evidence that native groups throughout Amazonia have been consuming acai palm fruit for more than 200 years, from the remarkably resilient Yanomami tribe in northwestern Brazil to numerous tribes living near the Amazon River estuary and its riverines.

In 2002 I commissioned a study to see if an acute dose of freeze-dried acai fruit pulp could hurt laboratory animals. At a single dose of 2,000 milligrams per kilogram it did not phase the animals or cause any adverse effects. This would be allometrically equivalent to humans consuming 140 grams all at once, or more than 50 times what one might usually eat in a day if taken as a dietary supplement.

In 2005 I commissioned a study to see if the freeze-dried acai (OptiAcai™) was mutagenic. There is evidence that mutagens are involved in tumor formation in humans and animals. The acai sample was found not to be mutagenic based on the bacterial reverse mutagenicity assay (using U.S. FDA compliant guidelines).

Oxidative Stress and Antioxidant Benefits

With the knowledge of its history of use as a food and scientific evidence of safety, comes the question of what might be its benefits.

At this time, epidemiological studies and clinical trials have determined that there is an inverse correlation between the intake of antioxidant-rich fruits and vegetables and the prevalence or occurrence of diseases such as cardiovascular disease, diabetes, cancer, inflammatory diseases and age-related diseases. Much of this has been pointed out in earlier chapters.

Dietary antioxidants are believed to be effective nutrients in the prevention of oxidative stress related diseases. Because acai fruit contains a number of proanthocyanidins, it may even do more than reduce the risk of diseases, it may delay some signs of aging. Oxidation causes the most visible sign of oxidative stress and aging on our skin. Hence, maintaining optimal antioxidant status makes sense. This may also explain why so many sunscreens now incorporate antioxidants into their formulations.

Oxidative stress can also be caused by the free radical species, peroxynitrite, known to damage the vascular endothelium, a process that if not kept in check can lead to atherosclerosis. Freeze-dried acai fruit has been shown to have antioxidant activity against peroxynitrite.

It is estimated that one percent of total oxygen consumed by an adult is converted to the free radical superoxide anion. The superoxide anion is believed to be the cause of other reactive oxygen species such as hydrogen peroxide, peroxynitrite and hydroxyl radicals (from hydrogen peroxide). Therefore, the superoxide scavenging capacity in the human body is the first line of defense against oxidative stress. Superoxide scavenging capacity in blood is a very important parameter in determining one's antioxidant status. Hence, freeze-dried acai fruit was subjected to the superoxide scavenging activity assay (SOD). Again to my surprise the SOD unit equivalent per gram were 1,614, more than three times greater than any food the lab had ever tested. The most studied source of superoxide scavenging activity in the diet had until this time been sprouted wheat, which ranged from 160 units to 500 units equivalent per gram. Essentially what this means is that consumption of freeze-dried acai fruit could reduce production of other free radicals owing to its potential to increase superoxide scavenging activity.

I have received reports from the United States, Puerto Rico, and Brazil of individuals claiming acai reduced the pain and discomfort associated with inflammatory conditions such as arthritis. Inflammation is a response of the immune system to chemical or physical assault, or resistance to pathogens. Although it is uncomfortable, even painful, inflammation is normally a part of healing. But in some chronic conditions, the inflammation is associated with debilitating diseases. It is now understood that one of the ways to reduce acute or chronic inflammation is to inhibit the activity of cyclooxygenase-2 (COX-2). Does acai have COX-2 inhibition capacity? Using a cyclooxygenase inhibitor assay that was developed to study samples of botanical origin, it was reported in 2006 that freeze-dried acai (OptiAcai) did have COX-2 inhibitory activity, but not as powerful as non-steroidal anti-inflammatory drugs (NSAIDs) or synthetic COX inhibitors, which have been reported to have an increased risk of adverse side effects. So there may be a basis for these anecdotal reports of benefit based on its inhibitory activity of COX-2.

It has also came to my attention during a trip to Brazil some years ago that acai is associated with an ability to decrease cholesterol levels in individuals with moderately elevated cholesterol, particularly those individuals needing to improve the ratio of low to high density lipoprotein-cholesterol (LDL-HDL cholesterol) to healthier levels. How might acai do this? This effect if real may be partially due to the amount of fiber in the pulp of freeze-dried acai fruit. In 2006 it was reported that freeze-dried acai fruit contains 84 percent of its fats as monounsaturated and polyunsaturated fatty acids, those "good" fats touted by so many health practitioners. Americans in particular, and a growing number of people around the world, consume too much saturated fat in comparison to these good fats, resulting in the ability of excess saturated fat to contribute to coronary vascular diseases. Hence, acai is a rich source of desirable fats good for the heart and circulation. The same 2006 also reported that freeze-dried acai contains phytosterols, specifically beta-sitosterol, campesterol, and sigmasterol all compounds known for their lipid lowering properties. These phytosterols are plant fats rather similar in structure to animal fat cholesterol. But they are different in chemical structure and thought by some researchers to be effective in the treatment or prevention of elevated cholesterol (hypercholesterolemia).

Two years earlier, the Universidade Federal Do Rio Grande do Norte in Brazil reported that proteins in acai pulp have high antitryptic activity and considerable inhibitory activity towards human salivary alpha-amylase. Determining salivary alpha-amylase (sAA) levels in humans is useful in measuring the degree of stress an individual is experiencing. An increase in sAA correlates with an increase in norepinephrine (also called noradenaline) and mirrors changes in cortisol levels that correlate with stress levels. Norepinephrine is produced by the adrenal gland and released into the bloodstream as part of the fight-or-flight response. Both a hormone and a neurotransmitter, norepinephrine is also released by nerve endings of the sympathetic nervous system resulting in an increase in the heart rate, blood pressure, and blood sugar level. Hence, the proteins in acai pulp, well preserved when freeze-dried, can contribute to coping with everyday stresses. This may explain why native Brazilians who consume acai with meals on a regular basis notice a difference within days of stopping their consumption of acai, as noted by a National Academy of Sciences survey done in Brazil in the late 1980's.

A new antioxidant assay developed at the University of California at Irvine, School of Medicine, called the Total Anti-oxidant (TAO) assay, can also determine a food's antioxidant capacity. The TAO is able to differentiate antioxidants into a "slow-acting" component, which includes complex organic antioxidants (e.g. phenolics) and a "fast-acting" or vitamin C-like component. The latter reflects the knowledge that vitamin C is more quickly excreted out of the body, and thereby loses its antioxidant activity much faster than other antioxidant sources.

The TAO assay results of freeze-dried acai (OptiAcai) clearly show that the antioxidant capacity of "slow-acting" antioxidants is stronger than that of the "fast-acting" antioxidants. This would mean that acai's antioxidants activity level against free radicals lasts longer. To ensure that a combination of slow and fast acting antioxidants is consumed to reduce excessive oxidative stress levels, it would seem prudent to combine vitamin C or fruits rich in vitamin C with acai, so as to benefit from both.

Studies yet to be published are also showing that acai can protect the cardiovascular system. One mechanism is by causing vasodilation of vessels carrying blood. Considering its high potassium content, that in itself probably contributes to this beneficial effect.

Chapter 8
Protection of Human Red Blood Cells

Human neutrophil cells are a type of white blood cell, specifically a form of granulocyte that contains tiny sacs of enzymes, that plays a major role in the body's defense against fungi, bacteria and viruses. The sacs of enzymes help the cell to kill and digest pathogens by a process called phagocytosis. If a person has too many neutriphils, a condition called neutrophilia, it is usually an indication that the person has an acute bacterial infection. If the person has a decreased proportion of neutophils in their blood, it might indicate they have a viral infection or are experiencing the effects of either chemotherapy or radiotherapy. In that case, it lowers their immunologic barriers to fungal and/or bacterial infection.

For these important reasons, a study of the effect of the freeze-dried acai on neutrophil cells seemed prudent, especially to see if it can reduce experimentally-induced oxidative stress – a condition linked to a wide range of diseases and conditions.

In a study reported in the *Journal of Food and Agricultural Chemistry* in 2006, blood samples were obtained from healthy volunteers. From these samples 100% neutrophil cells were harvested and used for evaluation of radical oxygen species (ROS) formation. Both acai-treated neutrophils cells and untreated neutrophil cells were exposed to hydrogen peroxide for 45 minutes, similar to what occur in the human body, resulting in oxidative stress from the body's release of hydrogen peroxide. This bioassay is commonly used to estimate the effectiveness of any given agent in terms of quenching hydrogen peroxide molecules. For this study the lab repeated the test several times to ensure the accuracy of the results.

The result of this study showed that pre-treatment of fresh human neutrophil cells resulted in significant reduction in ROS production. The formation of ROS was significantly inhibited, even at extremely low doses of freeze-dried acai down to a dilution of *one part per trillion*. In fact, it displayed a maximum effect at a concentration of 1-10 parts per trillion (ppt), which is at the physiologic levels that occur in the body, and has rarely been seen by any other natural compound. These results demonstrated a substantial inhibitory effect on the ROS formation in human neutrophil cells. The findings also indicate that the active anti-oxidant compounds in the freeze-dried acai tested are able to enter human cells in a fully functional form and perform oxygen quenching (scavenging) at extremely low doses. This may explain why just a few ounces of acai juice a day containing freeze-dried acai blended with other fruit juices has been reported to be of benefit for a wide range of oxidative stress related health conditions and diseases.

Chapter 9
Conclusion

Although acai fruit has a long history of traditional use in South America, I look forward to seeing more research done on this remarkable fruit from Amazonia. Only in this way can we eventually understand the full range of its nutritional benefits to humans.

What a string of discoveries: the highest Total ORAC of any food, the highest superoxide (SOD) scavenging of any food, able to quench superoxide, peroxynitrite and the hydroxyl and peroxyl radicals, with polyphenolics that are more powerful antioxidant compounds than found in any other berry. And in the laboratory it has been found to possess antioxidant activity when the freeze-dried powder is diluted down to one-part-per trillion. All of this, in addition to its nutritional composition, showing a complete complement of vitamins, minerals, amino acids, and healthy fatty acids, while low in sugar, and rich in fiber, makes you wonder why it took so long to discover it. Maybe it is because we have lost touch with the rest of the world, such as those natives in the Amazon who would not be surprised by all this excitement over a palm berry right in their back yard and found all over the Amazon.

Hence, knowledge related to acai can be summarized by the following points:

1) Only 5% of Americans consume at least 5 servings of fruits and vegetables per day. Less then 10% of these consume 9 or more servings. This highlights the need for sources of antioxidant-rich foods that are convenient, visually appealing, and taste good. For fruits this need is of even greater importance given how fast most fresh fruits perish, their high cost, and lack of year round availability.

2) Acai fruit consumption has a long history of traditional use traced to at least the late 18th century by Portuguese explorers, hardly making it a novel new food, although it is new to much of the world living outside of Brazil's borders.

3) The acai fruit is consumed by most natives living in the Amazon with virtually every meal of the day whenever the fruit is available. Studies have confirmed it is consumed at breakfast, lunch and dinner.

4) When prepared as a beverage, natives living in the Amazon consume up to 2 liters (64 fluid ounces) of fresh acai juice a day.

5) To capture the freshness of acai fruit, a proprietary freeze-dried acai has been used, produced in Brazil, to lock in the fruit's nutrients and phytochemical constituents. It is know by its tradename, OptiAcai. It was developed years ago for research because of the difficulty of transporting the fresh acai fruit to laboratories around the world.

6) The results of years of research performed by numerous laboratories and scientists with the freeze-dried powder have been published (see Schauss et al, 2006a and 2006b).

7) OptiAcai has been extensively studied laboratories because it is not an extract. It is the whole fruit pulp and skin quickly freeze-dried after harvesting so as to remove moisture and there by making it stable and low in microbiological load for study purposes. (An extract is a substance made by soaking an herb or fruit in a liquid that removes specific types of chemicals. Fresh freeze-drying allows maintenance of the natural potency of a food by preserving the biologically active constituents of the fresh plant without the use of chemicals, water or a combination of water and chemicals (e.g., hydroalcohol)).

8) A study of the use of acai fruit by natives living in Amazon has revealed that they feel it gives them energy without containing stimulants, such as caffeine. This may be due to the fruit's nutrient and phytochemical composition. No stimulants have been found in the fruit.

9) Research on freeze-dried OptiAcai has found that it has the highest Total Oxygen Radical Absorbance Capacity (T-ORAC), a combination of hydrophilic (water soluble) and lipophilic (fat soluble) scavenging (binding to the peroxyl free radical) activity in vitro of any fruit, vegetable or nut, tested for ORAC activity. The reported T-ORAC for OptiAcai is 1,026.9 micromole Trolox equivalent per gram. This is at least four times higher than any fruit, vegetable or nut in the world, that did not require chemical extraction to raise its antioxidant capacity.

10) Research on freeze-dried OptiAcai has found that it is far superior to spray-dried or frozen acai products. Spray-dried products are subjected to heat during processing and often are mixed with maltodextrin to stabilize them. Frozen acai products loss potency due to continuous degradation by enzymes that over time may affect the quality of the fruit in terms of its antioxidant capacity. For example, one frozen acai product was found to have a T-ORAC of 40, approximately 1/25th that of freeze-dried OptiAcai. This may be especially true when considering the distance needed to bring frozen product to market from the Amazon in large blocks that fill a shipping container, much of which is nothing more than water, and which obviously adds to both transportation cost and energy utilization.

11) Research on freeze-dried OptiAcai has found it has the highest lipophilic antioxidant activity of any fruit, based on the ORAC-lipophilic assay. This may be due to acai fruit's exceptionally high level of monounsaturated and polyunsaturated fatty acids.

12) Research on freeze-dried OptiAcai has found it has the highest hydrophilic antioxidant activity of any fruit, vegetable or nut, based on the ORAC-hydrophilic assay.

13) Research on freeze-dried OptiAcai has found it has the highest superoxide scavenging activity (SORAC) of any fruit, vegetable or nut. The reported SORAC activity is 1,614 units, nearly five times that of any other food known to have any superoxide scavenging activity in vitro. This unusually high SORAC activity may have significant benefit due to the role superoxide plays in forming highly reactive free radial oxygen species, such as the hydroxyl radical, which can be very destructive to cells.

14) Acai has a remarkable number of different flavonoids found in a wide range of foods associated with health giving benefits.

15) Acai is rich in anthocyanins and proanthocyanins a key group of polyphenolic compounds found to have antioxidant activity in vitro and in vivo.

16) Research on freeze-dried OptiAcai has found that it has anthocyanins that are 5 times more potent than the same class of anthocyanins found in other antioxidant-rich berries touted for their health giving properties.

17) Research on freeze-dried OptiAcai has found that it has "potent anti-inflammatory" activity in vitro.

18) Acai contains a whole range of essential vitamins, minerals, and trace elements.

19) Acai contains all of the essential and non-essential amino acids required for protein synthesis and other needs contributing to health maintenance.

20) Eighty percent (80%) of freeze-dried OptiAcai's fatty acids are monounsaturated and polyunsaturated fatty acids. This percentage is higher than that of olive oil or avocado oil.

21) Acai is a good source of soluble and insoluble fiber.

22) Compositional studies of the freeze-dried OptiAcai has determined it is very low in sucrose content (less than 1/10th of a gram per 100 grams) and simple sugars, lessening the risk of contributing to insulin resistance, with chronic use.

23) Research on freeze-dried OptiAcai has demonstrated that it is able to enter human cells in a fully functional form and perform oxygen quenching at extremely low doses, down to less than one part per trillion. This has been demonstrated using fresh human cells.

24) Acai has "organic" status as a food by nature because no pesticides, insecticides or herbicides are needed for the fruit to reach maturity twice a year. The palms that bear the fruit benefit from the natural biomass, rich in nutrients, the tropical forests of the Amazon region provide twice annually.

25) Acai is low in cholestrol. Research has found freeze-dried OptiAcai is 1.25% cholesterol.

26) Acai is low in sodium. Research has found freeze-dried OptiAcai is 0.25% sodium.

27) Acai contains numerous phytosterols, or plant fats, associated with health giving benefits.

28) Research on freeze-dried OptiAcai has been found to also have significant peroxynitrite radical scavenging activity based on its peroxynitrite radical scavenging capacity (NORAC) in vitro. The peroxynitrite radical is a strong oxidant and nitrating agent that damages DNA, proteins and other cellular structures, ascribed to the reaction of superoxide with nitric oxide, as well as carbon dioxide, in the body. The nitrogen dioxide and carbonate radical are believed to cause peroxynitite-related cellular damage.

29) Research on freeze-dried OptiAcai has been found to also have significant hydroxyl radical scavenging activity based on its Hydroxyl Radical Scavenging Capacity (HORAC) in vitro. The hydroxyl radical is highly reactive and short lived. It can damage virtually all types of macromolecules found in the body: amino acids, carbohydrates, nucleic acids (leading to mutations), fats (leading to lipid peroxidation). The only way to protect cells is the use of antioxidants formed in the body or obtained from antioxidant-rich foods.

30) Just a few grams of the freeze-dried OptiAcai can contribute toward meeting the estimated daily intake of 5,000 to 6,000 ORAC units from a variety of fruits and vegetables.

31) All of the above points have been published in peer review scientific journals.

As news of the nutritional value and antioxidant benefit of the acai fruit reaches across Amazonia, it will hopefully stimulate maximal protection of the precise palms that provide us the acai fruit berry. And by doing so, it is my hope that it will help protect and preserve this remarkable ecosystem that provides the world an estimated 20% of the world's oxygen supply, but also because it may hold yet another health giving food source or medicine. Already large areas of Brazil have fallen under the protection of regional and government agencies due the palms long-term economic value.

Finally, one has to marvel at the profound innate knowledge natives of the New World possessed for so many centuries in selecting this food as a significant part of their diet. Given the many nutritional and phytochemical attributes of the acai fruit recently discovered, is it any wonder why they consume this fruit with virtually every meal.

Maybe, just maybe, people with vision, will undertake a mission to bring this fruit to people around the world, and thereby allow others to benefit from its remarkable content so it can continue to serve as a guardian of the rain forest of the Amazon and protect all that lives and grows in and below it.

Acknowledgement

To the many scientists who contributed their time and effort to conducting studies on the composition and bioactivities of acai fruit. To Ken Murdock and K2A, LLC in Provo, Utah, for providing samples of freeze dried acai fruit pulp (OptiAcai™) for research. Special thanks goes to all the people who encouraged me to take a moment out of my research activities and write this book. To my wife, Laura, for proofreading the work and waiting for its completion, and to the wonderful people of Brasil (yes, that is the correct spelling), most of whom are engaged in a never ending battle to protect the rain forests and all the treasures it holds that gives life to this planet.

References

Anderson AB. Os nomes e usos de palmeiras entre uma tribo de indios Yanomama. Acta Amazonica, 1977; 7: 5-13.

Araújo, C. L.; Bezerra, I. W. L.; Dantas, I. C.; Lima, T. V. S.; Oliveira, A. S.; Miranda, M. R. R. A.; Leite, E. L.; Sales, M. P. Biological activity of proteins from pulps of tropical fruits. Food Chemistry, 2004; 85: 107-110.

Borbalan AM, Zorro L, Guillen DA, Barroso CG. Study of the polyphenol content of red and white grape varieties by liquid chromatography-mass spectrometry and its relationship to antioxidant power. Journal Chromatography, 2003; 1012: 31-8.

Bors W, Michel C, Stettmaier K. In: Flavonoids and Other Polyphenols (Methods in Enzymology Vol. 335); Packer, L. Ed. Academic Press: San Diego, 2001; p. 166-180.

Broschat TK, Meerow AW. Ornamental Palm Horticulture. University Press of Florida: Gainesville, 2000, pp. 61, 132.

Bushman BS, Phillips B, Isbell T, Ou B, Crane JM, Knapp SJ. Chemical composition of caneberry (Rubus spp.) seeds and oils and their antioxidant potential. Journal Agricultural Food Chemistry, 2004; 52: 7982-7987.

Cavalcante PB, Johnson D. Edible palm fruits of the Brazilian Amazon. In: Cavalcante: Edible Palm Fruits. Frutas Comestiveis da Amazonia II. Museu Goeldi: Belem, Brazil, 1974; and, Principes, 1977; 21: 91-102.

Chernela JM. The Wanano Indians of the Brazilian Amazon: A Sense of Space. University of Texas Press: Austin, TX, 1993, p. 112.

Durak I, Avci A, Kacmaz M, Buyukkocak S, Cimen MY, Elgun S, Ozturk HS. Comparison of antioxidant potentials of red wine, white wine, grape juice and alcohol. Curr Med Res Opin. 1999; 15:316-20.

Dyer AP. Latent energy in Euterpe oleracea. Universidad de Los Andes, Escuela de Ingenieria Forestal, Laboratorio de Bioenergia, LABONAC, Merida, Venezuela. Proceedings of the 9th Bioenergy Conference, Biomass Energy Environment, 1996, pp. 733-738.

Ellison D, and Ellison A. Betrock's Cultivated Palms of the World. Betrock Information Systems: Hollywood, FL, 2001, p. 110.

Ferreria AR. Viagem Filosofica: Pelas Capitanias do Grao Para, Rio Negro, Mato Grosso e Cuiaba, 1783-1792. Conselho Federal de Cultura: Rio de Janeiro, Brazil, 1971. (Drawing of Tanarana Indian gathering acai fruit.)

Henderson A, Galeano G, Bernal R. Field Guide to the Palms of the Americas. Princeton University Press, Princeton, NJ, 1995, p. 123-124, 284-285.

Huang, D, Ou B, Hampsch-Woodill M, Flanagan JA, Prior RL, Deemer EK. Development and validation of oxygen radical absorbance capacity assay for lipophilic antioxidants using randomly methylated beta-cyclodextrin as the solubility enhancer. Journal Agricultural Food Chemistry, 2002; 50: 1815-1821.

Huang, D, Ou B, Hampsch-Woodill M, Flanagan JA, Prior RL. High-throughput assay of oxygen radical absorbance capacity (ORAC) using a multichannel liquid handling system coupled with a microplate fluorescence reader in 96-well format. Journal Agricultural Food Chemistry, 2002; 50: 4437-4444.

Huang D, Ou B, Prior RL. The chemistry behind antioxidant capacity assays. Journal Agricultural Food Chemistry, 2005; 53: 1841-1856.

Iaderoza M, Baldini VLS, Draetta I dos S, Bovi MLA. Anthocyanins from fruits of acai (Euterpe oleracea, Mart) and jucara (Euterpe edulis, Mart). Tropical Sciences, 1992; 32: 41-46.

Jardim, M. A. G. and P. Y. Kageyama. Phenology of flowering and fruiting in a natural population of cabbage-palm (Euterpe oleracea Mart.) in the Amazon estuary. Boletim do Museu Paraense Emilio Goeldi Serie Botanica. 1994; 10: 77-82.

Jones DL. Palms Throughout the World. Smithsonian Institution Press: Washington, DC, 1995, p. 214.

Jordan M. In Brazil, a desparate struggle is waged over a salad garnish. The Wall Street Journal, March 25, 2002, p. 1.

Lescure JP, Castro A-de. Extractivism in central Amazonia. Bois et Forets des Tropiques. 1992; 231: 35-51.

Meerow AW. Betrock's Guide to Landscape Palms. Betrock Information Systems: Cooper City, FL, 1992, p. 46.

Meerow AW. Betrock's Guide to Landscape Palms, Ninth Edition. Betrock Information Systems: Hollywood, FL, 2004, p. 46.

Morell, V. The rain forest in Rio's backyard. National Geographic, 2004; 205(4): 3-22.

Muniz-Miret N, Vamos R, Hiraoka M, Montagnini F, Mendelsohn RO. The economic value of managing the acai plant (Euterpe oleracea Mar.) of the floodplains of the Amazon estuary, Para, Brazil. Forest Ecology Management, 1996; 87: 163-173.

Neto MAM, Alves JD, Oliveira de- EM. Anaerobic metabolism of Euterpe oleracea. II. Plant tolerance mechanism to anoxia. R Bras Fisiol Veg, 1995; 7: 47-51.

Ou B, Hampsch-Woodill M, Prior RL. Development and validation of an improved oxygen radical absorbance capacity assay using fluorescein as the fluorescent probe. Journal Agricultural Food Chemistry, 2001; 49: 4619-4626.

Ou B, Huang D, Hampsch-Woodill M, Flanagan JA, Deemer EK. Analysis of antioxidant activities of common vegetables employing oxygen radical absorbance capacity (ORAC) and ferric reducing antioxidant power (FRAP) assays: a comparative study. Journal Agricultural Food Chemistry, 2002; 50: 3122-3128.

Ou B, Hampsch-Woodill M, Flanagan J, Deemer EK, Prior RL, Huang D. Novel fluorometric assay for hydroxyl radical prevention capacity using fluorescein as the probe. Journal Agricultural Food Chemistry, 2002; 50: 2772-2777.

Ou B, Huang D, Hampsch-Woodill M, Flanagan JA. When east meets west: the relationship between yin-yang and antioxidant-oxidation. FASEB J, 2003; 17: 127-129.

Pannala AS, Rice-Evans C. In: Flavonoids and Other Polyphenols (Methods in Enzymology Vol. 335); Packer, L. Ed. Academic Press: San Diego, 2001; pp. 266-72.

Paula de- JE. Anatomia de Euterpe oleracea Mart. (Palma da Amazonia). Acta Amazonia, 1975; 5: 265-278.

Perricone N. The Perricone Promise: Look Younger, Live Longer in Three Easy Steps. Warner Books: New York, 2004.

Perricone, N. The Perricone Weight-loss Diet. Ballantine Books: New York, 2005.

Plotkin MJ, Balick MJ. Medicinal uses of South American palms. Journal Ethnopharmacology, 1984; 10: 157-179.

Pozo-Insfran D, Brenes CH, Talcott ST. Phytochemical composition and pigment stability of acai (Euterpe oleracea Mart.). Journal Agricultural Food Chemistry, 2004; 52: 1539-1545.

Prior RL, Hoang H, Gu L, Wu X, Bacchiocca M, Howard L, Hampsch-Woodill M, Huang D, Ou B, Jacob R. Assays for hydrophilic and lipophilic antioxidant capacity (oxygen radical absorbance capacity (ORACFL)) of plasma and other biological and food samples. Journal Agricultural Food Chemistry, 2003; 51: 3273-3279.

Rodriques de Areia ML, Miranda MA, Hartmann T. Memory of Amazonia: Alexandre Rodriues Ferreira and the Viagem Philosphica in the Captaincies of Grao-Para, Rio Negro, Mato Grosso, and Cuyaba. Museum of the Department of Anthropology, University of Coimbra, Portugal, 2003, plate 27.

Schauss, AG, Wu X, Prior RL, Ou B, Huang D, Owens J, Agarwal A, Jensen GS, Hart AN, Shanbrom E. Antioxidant capacity and other bioactivities of the freeze-dried Amazonian palm berry, Euterpe oleraceae Mart. (Acai). Journal Agricultural Food Chemistry, 2006a, 54(22): 8604-8610.

Schauss, AG, Wu X, Prior RL, Ou B, Patel D, Huangh D, Kababick JP. Phytochemical and nutrient composition of the freeze-dried Amazonian palm berry, Euterpe oleraceae Mart. (Acai). Journal Agricultural Food Chemistry, 2006b, 54(22): 8598-8603.

Schauss AG, Wu X, Ou B, Jensen GS, Agarwal A. High radical oxygen scavenging and antioxidant activity in freeze-dried Euterpe oleracea palm fruit pulp (OptiAcai). Federation Societies Experimental Biology Journal, 2006c; 20(4): A145.

Serafini M, Maiani G, and Ferro-Luzzi A. Journal of Nutrition 1998 128: 1003-7.

Serafini M, et al. Journal of Nutrition 2000 11: 585-90.

Shimkokomaki M, Abdala C, et al. Anatomy of Euterpe oleracea Mart. (Palmae of the Amazonia). Acta Amazonica, 1975; 5: 265-278.

Sick H. Birds in Brazil: A Natural History. Princeton University Press: Princeton, NJ, 1993, pp. 45, 447.

Skaper SD, et al. Free Radical Biology and Medicine 1997 22: 669-78.

Stevenson GB. Palms of South Florida. University Press of Florida: Gainesville, FL, 1996, p. 220.

Strudwick J, Sobel GL. Uses of Euterpe oleracea Mart. in the Amazon estuary, Brazil. In: The Palm--Tree of Life: Biology, Utilization and Conservation. Balick MJ [ed.] Advances in Economic Botany, Volume 6. New York Botanical Garden: Bronx, NY, 1988, pp. 225-253.

The Emerald Realm: Earth's Precious Rain Forests. National Geographic Society: Washington, DC, 1990.

Wada L, Ou B. Antioxidant activity and phenolic content of Oregon canberries? Journal Agricultural Food Chemistry, 2002; 50: 3495-3500

Wu X, Prior RL. Identification and characterization of anthocyanins by high-performance liquid chromatography-electrospray ionization-tandem mass spectrometry in common foods in the United States: vegetables, nuts, and grains. Journal Agricultural Food Chemistry, 2005; 53: 2010-3113.

Wu X, Prior RL. Systematic identification and characterization of anthocyanins by HPLC-ESI-MS/MS in common foods in the United States: fruits and berries. Journal Food Agricultural Food Chemistry (in press).

Wu X, Prior RL, Schaich K. Standardized methods for the determination of antioxidant capacity and phenolics in foods and dietary supplements. Journal Agricultural Food Chemistry, 2005; 53: 4290-4302.

Wu X, Beecher GR, Holden JM, Haytowitz DB, Gebhardt SE, Prior RL. Lipophilic and hydrophilic antioxidant capacities of common foods in the United States. Journal Agricultural Food Chemistry, 2004; 52: 4026-4037.

Wu X, Gu L, Holden J, Haytowitz DB, Gebhardt SE, Beecher G,Prior RL. Development of a database for total antioxidant capacity in foods: preliminary study. Journal Food Composition Analysis, 2004; 17: 407-422.